Before You Go,

Life Advice for the Rising Generation

by Mr. H

Goodbye

Anyone who's been a teacher or parent knows the feeling you get when a kid moves to the next stage in life whether it's graduation, college, moving out, moving away or getting married. It's a cocktail of emotions: happiness at seeing them succeed, excitement and hope for what they will accomplish in the upcoming years, sadness to see this chapter in their life close, and anxiety for the challenges that lay ahead for them.

The odds are, you've seen a significant amount of those challenges firsthand. You feel a small sense of helplessness knowing that there is only so much more you can do to impact their life. You can see around the corners they are heading towards but only *they* can walk around them. You can make all the mistakes so that they don't have to but they will inevitably have to learn some of those the same way you did; the hard way. You're not just instructing a child or a teen or a young adult. You're helping to build a human being; hopefully a *moral, productive, sociable* and *strong* one.

I found this to be especially concerning my first year of teaching. As a parent, I have every day and night to instruct my children on the path God is setting for them. At the parochial school that I've taught at, I only have an hour a day with each student to teach them the criteria and to play a small role in shaping them into the people God made them to be. The end of the school year sends a fresh class of graduating young men and women out the door and into the world beyond. In that moment I realized how little I was actually able to teach them in the grand scheme of things. I look at the adversities, dangers and foolish roads that lie ahead of them and want them all to find their way safely to the other side of full adulthood as outstanding citizens.

This book is meant to give all of those former students of mine, and any more out there who are exiting out different sets of doors than mine, a few more nuggets of wisdom. I have to admit, I don't have that many to give out to begin with. The few I *do* have, I struggle at putting into practice every bit as much as the next guy. But for what it's worth, I try. I'm no expert or authority on anything in life, but God has put me around some people who are. I've tried to learn from them.
Whoever you are, wherever you are, I hope you can use some or all of these pieces of advice and make your life just a little more meaningful. I hope there's something in this book that helps you to grow and mature, to see the best in others and that brings out the best in you. As a Christian, I hope this book gives a little bit of the light God gave to me because what good does having His gifts do if you're not willing to share them? I wish you the best of luck on your journey down the road He has for you.

I pray for you and your success.

God bless,

Mr. H

Mental Frameworks

Let's start with what a mental framework is and why it matters for you to care what they are. A **mental framework** is a baseline thought that precedes or colors every other thought or notion you have. Mental frameworks are like a combination of lenses that you see the world with. No matter what you look at, they affect how you see it and can even obscure or clarify what it is you see. Think of a yellow tinted pair of construction glasses. You can still see everything when you're wearing them. But no matter what you look at, it will have a yellow quality to it. It can help you see into the water a little better by cutting the glare or can hide that yellow golf ball lying in the grass.

Here's a real world example:

Two men, John and Henry, can get cut off in traffic. John was raised to be gracious with people's mistakes. He was taught by his parents to understand that a day's outcome is only as good or bad as his decision to make it so. He sees inconveniences as small parts of a day he's already blessed to be alive for. Henry was raised quite differently. He was raised to see the day like a math equation: negative things subtracted against positive ones on a scale. If a greater number of bad incidents happened than good incidents, the day is ruined for Henry. Each day is a desperate race to make sure the equation lands on the positive side or his day wasn't worth getting out of bed for.
Who do you think will respond with more tact and maturity based on their mental framework? John will most likely go about his day, driving on to his destination

without a second thought. He may honk his horn politely to avert the potential danger of a collision and turn this event into a small joke at work but beyond that, the situation has little effect on his life. Henry, you can imagine, will most likely devolve into antics commonly seen during a road rage incident. He'll seek to even the scales and get retribution from the offending vehicle. If you have any doubts, YouTube is full of evidence of these men and women who lose control on the road because their mental framework was twisted. The consequences can be disastrous.

Our mental frameworks will determine what our goals are because they can change what we think is possible, probable or inevitable. Sometimes all it takes is a suggestion of what is possible. Other times we have to see it to believe it. But *how* we think will most often determine whether we're even willing to *try*. If you want to improve your life, you have to start understanding how you think and asking yourself if the way you're thinking encourages you to operate at the highest level and to live your life joyfully and productively.

So let's go over some helpful ones.

You are your habits

The little things you do everyday will determine the vast majority of your life. They define what your priorities are, what you will dedicate your time, money and resources to and how successful you will be in any particular long term endeavor.

If you work out once a month for three hours straight but every other day you plop yourself down on the couch and watch your favorite show on HBO Max, then you're not a person who works out. You're a person who sits and watches TV. If you sleep in for nine days then wake up early on the tenth day, you're not an early riser. You're a late waker.

Success is built in miniscule increments by comparison of where you start with where you want to be.

There's an old comical question that goes:

"How do you eat an elephant?"

to which the reply is:

"One bite at a time."

You may feel like you made incredible progress one day and maybe you did. But when you compare it to the total road ahead, it's just a tiny step. It's easy to get discouraged when you know this fact. That's why it's important to make successful habits as early as possible. If you're not feeling motivated to do something one day, your habits that you've built up can help you default to doing it anyway. Start early and do it consistently.

This will make it a habit.

And you *are* your habits.

Assume ignorance over malice

It's a small world and it gets a whole lot smaller if you go around thinking every bad thing someone does to you was because of a grudge or hatred or bigotry or evil intent.

When you've lived longer than five or so years outside of a school setting you begin to realize something: everyone is ignorant...even you. We all have blind spots and limited areas of knowledge and consciousness. We don't quickly see other people's experiences and we relate to them even more slowly.

So when that guy cuts you off in line or your teacher or boss calls you out for something that a peer just did five minutes ago, don't assume they have it out for you. People have way too much going on in their lives to have space in their heads to worry about you. You're just not that important, my friend.

But that's a good thing!

Think of it this way: Could you possibly have the mental bandwidth to think about every other human being alive and also strategize their ultimate demise?
I doubt it. Everyone else is the same way.

So can people be ignorant and self-centered and sometimes a little rude?

Yep.

But is the whole world plotting your downfall one small move at a time?
Nope.

So take a deep breath, assume that most bad things that happen to you could've just as easily happened to the guy next to you and get on with your day.

You'll be happier, you'll sleep easier, you'll be a heck of a lot more fun to be around and most importantly, you won't go burning bridges after every inconvenience.

Assume ignorance over malice.

You don't know what you don't know

Have you ever heard the term "Black Swan Event"?

The term refers to an event that occurs despite knowledge to the contrary. The whole world understood that black swans did not exist...right up until 1697 when one was discovered in the wild. Since that fateful day, we have used the term 'black swan event' to refer to a highly impactful event that could not have been foreseen with the knowledge at the time. The world was confident that the earth was the center of the universe until one day it wasn't. Everybody knew that sailing across the Atlantic from Europe was suicide, until intrepid explorers proved otherwise.

Our knowledge is limited to our time.

The primary point of this topic is **humility**. Life is full of unexpected events on a personal and a societal level. Despite our best efforts to stay informed or in the loop or doing our own research, we cannot possibly know everything. Even with the world of knowledge at our fingertips in the form of an iPhone or Android, there is too much to know in the world and not enough lifetime to learn it. Most of the time, we don't even know what it is we need to know. We're explorers without a map, compass or destination in mind.

The most successful people in life understand this and approach life with humility, trying to learn as much from everyone around them as possible. Everyone has areas of expertise. Everyone knows something we don't. The smartest man in the world doesn't have one billionth of

the combined knowledge of your hometown so keep that in mind before strutting around, self assured that you know more than people because of your education, your pedigree, your training or your accolades.
You should see this as a relief. It'd be a bummer to know everything in the world. Imagine that kind of pressure. I sure wouldn't want it. So when you go out into the world, do it with a humble understanding that everyone has something they can offer you. You can be surprised by anyone at any time with knowledge that could change your entire world.

This makes life so much more exciting, by the way. Humanity becomes a treasure hunt of wisdom and, with a little conversational skill, you can start knowing just a little bit more of what you don't know.

Life is a network of relationships so don't burn bridges

This one is pretty self explanatory in my opinion but, since 'you don't know what you don't know', I'll explain further just in case.

There's a game that people play called 'Six Degrees of Kevin Bacon'. In the game, a random actor is called out and through a connection of different films, directors and projects, you can associate just about anybody with iconic Hollywood actor Kevin Bacon.

So what does this have to do with advice for success in life?

This game gives a little wink to a truth that exists in all of our lives. No matter how distant you think a person may be from you, you never know just how connected they may be to you. We all have family, friends, associates, coworkers, classmates, former classmates, teachers, teammates, coaches, neighbors and fellow parishioners that we see everyday. We travel all over the community, the state, the country and the world. And now, in the age of social media, this concept has been pushed to it's absolute limits. We are connected as a society in so many ways. That's by design. People are made for communities. We thrive on positive relationships and operate at our best when our life and work are contributing to the lives of others.

Yes, introverts, I'm even talking about us.

So when you get angry at someone or your boss pushes you just a little too far, as much as you'd like to tell them off, keep something in mind: it's a small world.

The guy you insult today could be interviewing you tomorrow or the girl who you made feel terrible about herself could be your future wife's best friend. The woman you cut off in traffic could be your nurse the next time you're in the hospital and the guy you called a 'stupid hick' online could be the man who drives by when you're on the side of the road with a flat tire.

Our responsibility as adults in this world is to make it a happier, healthier, more morally based place than the one we inherited. You can't do that by throwing metaphorical grenades into every interaction. One drop of poison in that network of relationships can tarnish years of careful building.

People are also **memetic**, meaning that we mirror others who we are around. The positivity we feed into the world will inspire more of itself.The opposite is also true. You are responsible for building the culture you want to live in. Small acts of negativity can last a long time in people's memory so be careful how you treat others. You can disagree with people and avoid associating with others. You can be direct and to the point and not take much effort in sugar coating things. But always be respectful, even when you're not getting much in return.

As the old timers say, "What goes around, comes around" so don't burn bridges.

Be more afraid of who you'll become if you lie than the consequences of telling the truth

Fear is a powerful motivator. We shouldn't live our lives according to it but it's a helpful tool for survival and can lead us to excel when put in its proper context.

So with that in mind, let me tell you what the consequences of the truth will be.
You will suffer. Sometimes in small ways, other times tremendously. Telling your dad that you stole his liquor to throw a party while he was out of town could get you in a world of pain. He could do what my own dad would've done and whip your butt. You could be grounded for months at a time and his trust in you could be hurt for years to come. The hurt can be monumental. But you will still be intact as a person. Some of that trust will remain because you were forthright about what you did when asked. Your words still have value. Telling your mom you snuck out or your teacher that you cheated on the exam could bring similar trials. But facing them with the truth at your center will leave your world as a whole, unchanged.

With that being said, one lie can bring so much misery into your life.

The moment you tell a lie a multitude of things begin to happen. First, you have now become morally compromised. You are no longer an honest person. You may continue to be seen as one by the outside world but on the inside, you have now corrupted a part of yourself. You lose a vital aspect of your life that we all need to stay sane which is *reality*. When we invent a fiction, the first thing our minds do is attempt to reconcile that with the reality that contradicts it. This can force us to melt reality with unreality. We justify immoral behavior. We invent more things to bolster the original false claim. We begin to try and convince others of the falsehood as well and sometimes even encourage them to take part in the fantasy. We even begin to fool ourselves. We begin to see honesty as a threat and suspect others of the same moral corruption we now suffer from. The world becomes darker. It isn't the same world. You've walked through a door that isn't quickly returned from. Some people feel guilt and shame. Others don't. But no one feels morally well and spiritually sound after telling a falsehood. No one is made better from a lie.

In the end, your life is far better off living the world of truth and reality over lies and fiction. The temporary pain of truth is nothing compared to the monumental suffering of a single lie.

So, be more afraid of who you will become if you lie than the consequences of telling the truth.

Proper Preparation Prevents Poor Performance

Ah yes, the wonderful five P's of success.
The boy scouts have a shorthand phrase for this, "Be Prepared".
Prepared for what?
It doesn't matter. Just be ready.

Most of the problems you will encounter in life could be solved by giving the problem its proper attention and readiness beforehand. When our day starts to go wrong, proper planning creates a margin of error to give us room for things outside of our control. That could be packing an extra shirt, filling up on gas the night before school, carrying a flashlight in your bag or getting your concealed handgun license.

Consider Frank, who needs to get to work on time. He leaves with just enough time to get there according to the map. But he hits some unexpected traffic. Seeing that he's now primed to be late, he begins to speed to make up the time but keeps getting stuck behind cars going the speed limit or slower. Frustrated, he veers around each, cutting lanes to do so and gets pulled over. When he arrives half an hour late and gets reprimanded by his boss, Frank heatedly protests that he couldn't help that he got stuck in traffic because there are lots of incompetent drivers and a cop who was a jerk. But all of this could've been avoided had he prepared some margin room for traffic and road problems in his departure from home. He could've been prepared to be at work fifteen minutes early. Now he's thirty minutes late.

Proper planning prevents poor performance.

You need silence
Use it to your advantage

It's no secret that our world is too loud.
Our attention spans are too short.
We're too easily distracted.
Our lives are a blur.

When your room is too cluttered and messy you take out the trash. When your desk is chaotic, you clear it up. If your yard looks like crap, you clear out the dead brush and trim and cut it. The same logic applies to our lives. We can't have nonstop noise polluting our ears. We need intentional moments of silence to think, to create, to focus and to recharge.

Even when we are around people, silence can be a good thing. Sitting in peaceful contentment of someone's company without words can do wonders for a friendship or relationship. It establishes comfort and security. The same goes for a spouse. Sometimes, words just get in the way.

We can get our most profound thoughts, artistic revelations and breakthrough ideas during moments of absolute silence. One surprising note on this essential element is that most of us don't even realize how necessary it was until we get it. Our lives are blurred by reverberating noise and as soon as we step into pure silence, it can be like looking through water once the ripples disappear.

The greatest saints and thinkers of all time from Saint Thomas Aquinas and Saint Dominic to Steve Jobs and Elon Musk will readily admit to the practical uses of silence for their success. Sometimes, you just have to face your thoughts head on. There is no profession or age that is excluded from the need to experience a reduction in external noise because we're *all* thinking creatures.

From musicians and painters to plumbers and lawyers, we all need silence.

So use it to your advantage.

You need a base
Faith
Family
Community
Everything Else

Let's get dark for just a second.

You're going to die.
You're going to suffer.
You're going to suffer a lot.
That's part of living in this world.

That wasn't so bad was it?

There's an old saying that, "He who has a strong enough '**why**' can endure any '**what**'"
No matter what you are suffering from, if you have a powerful enough reason to push through that pain, you will continue living and thriving on a mental and spiritual level. The best evidence of this is in the stories of the saints I grew up learning about.

Saint Laurence was burned alive on a griddle by the Roman Empire for his Christian faith. While smelling his charring flesh, he looked out at his tormentors and nodded to his blackened skin saying, "You can turn me over. I'm done on this side". He's burning alive and he cracks a joke as if he's a steak! This was a man who had everything to gain from saying a couple of meager words. All he had to do was deny his faith and he could've had a quick and painless death. There was no material need to suffer. But he didn't live for comfort. He didn't live for wealth. He didn't even live to avoid pain. He had priorities that were larger and more purposeful than what the world could offer.

In your life you will lose much of what you take for granted. Tragedy can strike in a moment. So what you take security in and what your foundation in life is cannot be something that is easy to take away.

Start with your **faith**. This is something that cannot be broken, injured, stolen or confiscated. No government can touch it and cancer cannot kill it. It will feed your heart and soul every day of your life and give you strength when you lose everything else, even the next thing on this list.

Your **family** is your tightest human connection in your life. They have the most tangible and real bond to you and it's more than personal interest that keeps them tethered to you. We're not just morally attached. We are biologically driven to remain close to our family and to protect and support them. It's absurd how backwards we've gotten this in society. It's nothing short of creepy to see influencers and talking heads on television, Hollywood, and social media advocate for friction and distancing within a family. Friends, associates and acquaintances can be fickle. You can live in adoration from them one minute and scorn and rejection the next. Your family, with rare exceptions, will be the one door open to you when every other door is closed.

The next priority in your life is your **community**. Trust can be earned through familiarity and mutual commitment. The people in your neighborhood, church and local community will most likely share more in common with you than not. They have a stake in the success of your surroundings because they share them as well. They see your habits and routines and usually begin to base some of their own routines on yours without realizing it. Get to know your neighbors and other members of your community. Take care of those around you on a small scale and those spheres of influence will grow and strengthen. This is how you can *truly* change a nation. Bringing food to a fellow church goer after their spouse dies or mowing your neighbor's lawn when he's sick will do far more to create tangible change than rallies, protests, riots and social media posting.

Build your life from the ground up with a solid foundation and sturdy pillars.

Your faith is your foundation.
Your family is your set of pillars.
Your community is the roof over your head.

After that, let everything else in this world get in line.

Don't judge the past by today's standards

It's easy for us to be prideful as human beings and to become "chronological snobs" as the author C.S. Lewis put it.

We look at great men and women of the past and disregard them because their choices and lifestyles don't line up with ours. But all the while, we stand on their shoulders and take for granted the benefits they created for us.

A person's contributions to the world are not dependent on the views or sentiments of later generations. It's an impossible task to judge a man outside of the time he lived in. History moves slowly and people, as imperfect as we are, can only move within the time and space that we find ourselves in. A thousand years ago, public torture was not only acceptable for criminals but encouraged and treated like a sporting event. Two hundred years ago, a vast majority of the world didn't think twice about slavery or its morally devastating effect on humanity. Great men and women who did more for society than you or I ever have owned slaves.
Does this make slavery good?
Absolutely not.
But does this make those great men and women evil?
No.

Many of the American founding fathers owned slaves and began to slowly come to the realization that freedom was meant for all men, not just the ones who signed that world changing document. President Washington's personal writings describe his internal struggle to reconcile his ownership of men and women and his advocacy for freedom. History proves Washington to be a great man, living in a time that overwhelmingly believed something evil; that some human beings could be bought and sold. It was a belief he was raised with as a child and was in the very air he breathed from infancy to his dying breath. The miracle of our nation is that despite this overwhelming corruption of society across the entire world, his heart and mind still began to change towards freedom for **all** men.

You will be hard pressed to find a single great man or woman who didn't have vices congruent with the times whether that was conquest, drinking or insensitivity towards certain groups. Greatness is not a value based on time but of contribution that supersedes time. Objective morality never changes across the ages but history is made of broken men who were used to advance God's perfect vision. If you want to criticize those that came before you, roll your sleeves up, get some sweat on your brow and accomplish more than what they did.

How many people today spit on Washington for owning slaves but wear Nike shoes made from sweatshops filled with deprived children? How many people denigrate Thomas Jefferson on their iPhones for owning slaves while ignoring the fact that their phone batteries contain cobalt from mines worked by slave labor in Congo and the phone was assembled in Chinese sweatshops?
How many people recoil at the inhumane treatment of humans through slavery over a hundred years ago but dehumanize the tiniest and most vulnerable humans among us today: innocent babies? No one hears their cry and their right to life is considered forfeit based on all of the *same* arguments used by slave owners in the nineteenth century. How much have we really changed? Would you *really* be so different if you lived in their time?

Remember, one day your own record will be on the dock to be judged despite values of society continuing to change. One day your posts, comments, photos and lifestyle will fall under the same merciless gaze of a society that has moved on beyond your own values. What do **you** accept today that could be morally atrocious in a hundred years?

Be humble.

Don't judge the past by today's standards.

Ask *not* "can I have..."
Ask "how can I earn..."

As a coach, this mental framework hits close to home.

Everybody wants something.
Not everyone is willing to earn it.
Odds are that there's something that you want right now
and if that's the case, there's just as big a chance that
there's someone you have to go through to get it.

If it's a raise, you have to go through a boss.

If it's a starting spot on the football team, you have to go
through the coach.

If it's an extra credit assignment for a higher grade, you
have to go through your teacher.

So what makes you different from the other student who
wants an 'A' or player that wants the spot or worker that
wants the raise?
How do you stand out from the others in line who want
the exact same thing?

If all you do is ask for what you want then there really isn't
a difference. You need to distinguish yourself. To do that
you have to find out what you're missing; what it is that
you need to get what you want. Who better to tell you than
the decision maker for you getting it?

When you ask a coach, "how can I earn the starting spot"
you're accomplishing a couple things at once. First, you're
getting vital information you need for how you must

improve to get the spot. There's always a reason you don't have what you want. Getting that answer is half the battle. Second, you're sending a clear message to your coach that you *want* to get better, you're *open to his feedback* and you're *willing* to make an adjustment. This is a much more effective strategy to success than just asking to be given something. It sends a message of work ethic over entitlement, determination over desperation, action over words.

Ask not "can I have…" but "how can I earn…"

No one cares about your goals more than you do
Quit expecting them to

This is a simple message for everyone in every walk of life: your personal goals belong to *you* and *you alone.*

Everyone is the main character in their own story and we're all motivated to go after our goals before all others. So when you want to become the valedictorian of your campus, don't expect others to move mountains to make that happen for you.

Your teachers want you to succeed but they have their own goals. Your parents want you to be happy and successful but they also have other goals they are trying to achieve, even for you sometimes. Your friends are striving for their own visions and the rest of the world is doing the same.

Don't expect things to just fall into place and don't anticipate favors or breaks. Assume that all the work will need to be done yourself and make the conscious decision that what you want is important enough to do each and every painful task to accomplish it. If some lucky breaks or favors happen along the way, that's nice. But don't be dispirited or distraught if they don't.
Sometimes your goals may even be in direct conflict with your friends and peers. Don't take it personally if they work against you. Be determined to meet your goal regardless of the influence of others.

That may require more of you than of them.
Perhaps you didn't come from wealth or you have a lower IQ. Perhaps your parents are divorced or you suffered a

violent trauma. The heights of success for you may have more rungs on the ladder to get there. Trying to cut down others or whining about your lot in life won't help you get any higher or further in life.
Having fortitude and control of your intentions and actions will.

So set your goals and don't expect others to care about them as much as you do.

Define success before you chase it

People drift with the current under normal circumstances. We do it physically, mentally and emotionally. As a Catholic, I can even vouch that we do it spiritually.

When we set goals for success and don't have a specific set of markers for what it is we're trying to do, we will inevitably follow the path of least resistance.

To use an example, think of Chad, who's going to the weight room today. He has no goal of what he wants to achieve in the gym so he doesn't know what workouts will be effective. He tries a couple exercises for a few repetitions and then stops when he's tired or uncomfortable. He runs on a treadmill for a few minutes until he feels sweaty. He spends more time on his phone than with the iron and when he leaves, he is no stronger or more athletic than when he entered. All he really did was change his geography from home to a gym for an hour or so.

Now picture Amy, a young lady who enters the gym right as Chad is leaving. She knows she wants stronger legs that can beat her previous squat max of two hundred fifteen pounds and more defined abdominals and wants to trim a little bit of the belly fat that's hiding them. She walks over to the racks and starts building up repetitions on squats and works other leg routines to strengthen each part of her legs, focusing on adding more reps or more weight than the last time she was at the gym. Then she does ab exercises, making sure to do an extra five reps than the previous time she was at the gym. She walks out feeling exhausted, sweaty and sore, but far closer to the success that she clearly defined.

Attempting to gain success is meaningless if you don't know precisely *what* that looks like. For some people that can mean having zero debt in their life. Others can see it as being in excellent health with no sick days on that business year. Others can consider success as having a wife and children. Others may settle on just having someone to date and share their life with. We all have to find our way to the truth of what the ideal is and then pursue it relentlessly. But we are no more successful in achieving it without a definition than we would be navigating without a map and compass. (Or phone with GPS).

So get your target set up and define success before you chase it.

You are the summit of your entire family
Don't embarrass them

There's plenty of debate about the origin of human life.

Despite those that say we've been around for hundreds of thousands of years or just a few thousand, I think we can all agree that before us there came many, many, *many* generations of men and women. This amasses, for each one of us, thousands of individuals on thousands of different tracks of life producing billions of stories and moments to lead us where our own two feet now stand. Whether you're religious or not, that's quite a miracle of chance that you, and all the characteristics that make you up, exist.

That's like winning the lottery, my good friend.
It looks like we both have.

That makes me quite happy to think about. It also adds a sense of responsibility. Men died to get us here. Women took chances and made supreme sacrifices. Men faced dark days and terrible doubts and threats and fought for us to exist. Women showed courage and endured impossible hardships and daunting levels of pain for you and I to be where we are now.

Our family name, despite any off color stories about it, is actually the story of endurance and life against impossible odds. That carries a weight of responsibility for us.
What we say and do; what we don't say and don't do, can determine whether those thousands and thousands of years were futile or worth all of those generations of strife. That doesn't mean we have to be world conquerors and warriors that rival the great legends. But ask yourself,

"What would my ancestors think of me? What would they think of their own life as a result of seeing mine?" When someone makes a sacrifice for us, we should see to it that they didn't waste their time and effort. That goes for small favors from friends to a chance at life from our predecessors.

Be mindful of what you say and what you do. Be worthy of the name you were given and the history it took to create you.

Remember that you are the summit of your entire family so wherever they are in life (or the hereafter), don't embarrass them.

All men are called to fatherhood
All women are called to motherhood

Before the popular culture pitchfork mob comes after me, let me explain.

A vast majority of men and women are called to be biological or adoptive parents. We wouldn't exist as a species otherwise and even beyond that, this concept ties in quite neatly with the previous mental framework.

If millions of people struggled and suffered over thousands of generations to bring you into the world, it would be absurd for you to boldly claim that their bloodline should end on a whim you have.

On a smaller scale, that would be like inheriting a mansion and burning it to the ground because there was a spec of dust on the kitchen floor. Talk about a major fumble.

But what about those who cannot have children or truly are not called to have children such as religious clergy, people with same sex attractions or other special cases?

You are *still* called to fatherhood and motherhood; just in a different way.

We are *all* called to take our wisdom of experience and pass it along to younger generations. It is how we have come so far as a human race. Over all the years of our existence, we have created a largely unbroken chain of information, culture and tradition that has produced wonderful and tremendous things with the guiding hand of God.

That all starts with the acceptance that we cannot just let all that we have learned and experienced die with us.

We need a prodigy.

For most, this will be in the form of actual marriage and children. This is an amazing experience that I can attest to myself as a father. Like any other form of mentorship, it is incredibly difficult at times and has no shortage of pain and heartache. Their suffering becomes yours. But their triumphs and joys become yours as well. And trust me, young minds find *so much* to take joy in.

For others, this may come in the form of education such as teachers, youth pastors, private lesson providers, coaches and camp counselors. While these positions don't have the same connection as a mother and father, they are incredibly powerful and influential areas of a child's life in which you have the ability to pass on your knowledge of relevant material to the next generation. I can also attest to this as a teacher and coach.

For the few that simply struggle with working with children at all, there is still a calling to mentor others. If you are in this group, there are others around you who are younger and less experienced at something that you can help. At your job, there are no doubt others who are younger and less experienced. They need a mentor or guide to help show them the way. There may be neighbors who are struggling to adjust to the area or youngsters in your social group or club or church who need your guidance. Help them. Fulfill your calling.

We are all called to parenthood or mentorship.

Life is a paradox
The more you give to others,
the bigger you become

Love is a central pillar of what makes us human.

The ability to actively work for the good of someone other than ourselves, meaning the **true** definition of love, is what allows us to flourish. It's important to love ourselves too but the prime attribute of love is selflessness. There is no worthwhile area of your life that will not be improved by seeking to make others better off and serving others before yourself on an individual level.

Society sees people who do this differently. People who are truly selfless may not always be liked. Sometimes they are even hated and despised. But they make the greatest impacts for good in this world and their words and deeds have more weight than those of a selfish person. Think of the greatest men and women in history. They all gave far more than they ever received; yes, even some of those "dirty rotten billionaires".

What you will also find when you begin to put this in practice is that the more you give to others, the more *joy* you take in doing it. Your life means a whole lot less when you live for yourself. When you live for others, your world grows with each person you choose to serve.

The good your selflessness does will spread like a wildfire, even in ways that you cannot immediately see. It's not about instant gratification but creating a current of care in our culture.

And you can give so much more than money. You can give attention to someone who feels abandoned and alone. You can give advice to someone who is lost in their way and needs direction. You can give wisdom to a younger person who needs a friend of experience. You can give connections to someone who has no lifeline to call. You can give laughter to a person who hasn't had a reason to smile in weeks or more. The possibilities to give to others are all around us and in abundant supply. You just need the will to look around and love the people you see.
It's a strange little fact of life but it's verifiably true.

The more you give to others, the bigger you become.

Loving someone doesn't mean affirming everything they say, do or believe

Speaking of love, we need to talk about it a little longer. I have a hunch I'll take some hate for this one.

Love is not a Hollywood feeling.

It's not sunny days, a quickened heartbeat or a swell of Hallmark music before a Hollywood kiss. It's not fireworks or passion. You don't 'fall into love' or 'out of love' and it's not a warm and fuzzy sensation.

Sorry.

Love, as it has been understood for thousands of years, is the **intentional working for the good of someone else**. Love is a verb. It requires will and action.

As long as we're living in reality, we can assume that there are some things that are good and some things that aren't. That's called objective truth. So when you love someone, that doesn't mean agreeing with everything they say, supporting everything they do and not giving any resistance to them.

If I love my mother, I'm not going to support her if she decides to drain a bottle of Jack Daniel's and hit the highway for a midnight drive.
If I love my children, I won't affirm their belief that they can fly by throwing them off the roof of my house.
If my wife loves me, she won't stand by and do nothing if I decided one day to pick up robbing banks as a new line of work (only if this whole writing thing doesn't work out).
As the old book says, love is patient, love is kind, etc, etc.

What it doesn't say is "love is indulgent" or "love is enabling".

It's inevitable that the people around us who we care about will sometimes do destructive things. We're imperfect creatures. It's important to remember that if someone is doing something that can harm themselves or others, your love for them *obligates* you to do everything in your power to stop them. And they should do the same when you fall from grace. Perhaps this advice is ill suited for professional success or even financial success.

But in the areas it matters most, this mental framework can help save the ones you love, and possibly even you.

There is no problem you can fix by hating people

People are not problems.

People can create problems.

When you understand this you will begin to realize how much more can be accomplished by focusing your energy on attacking problems and trouble rather than people and personalities.

People create problems because we are broken by nature and are prone to sin and error. But the problems that we create, once they leave us, become separate and tangible things in the world that must be dealt with. Hating the person who creates the problem may feel good for your righteous anger but it is impotent against the problem itself.

Even if your anger is justified at the person who started the issue, any effort and energy you spend on hating that person for the original mistake does nothing to deal with the obstacle that's now in front of you.

Hatred itself is not always a bad thing. We have this feeling of anger and hatred for a reason. It is an inner calling towards justice and righteousness. God placed it in us for a reason. But like a power saw, it is only meant to be used on *things,* not *people.*

It is okay to hate things such as child abuse, murder, disease and corruption. It's not okay, and solves nothing to hate the abuser, the murderer, the sick or the corrupt.

This is a huge undertaking and a radical shift for many if not most people.

But it's not exactly a new thought. Two thousand years ago, Jesus of Nazareth instructed his followers of this same concept. Many took it quite harshly. A considerable amount of them walked away on the spot. But that line of thinking, to hate the sin and to love the sinner has proven to be a sustainable mental framework for two millenia.

We have a limited amount of hours and energy and allowing any of it to be siphoned away on attacking people is time and energy not spent on actually getting things done.

So as hard as it may be sometimes, especially when it concerns a topic that is significantly emotional for you, don't waste yourself by hating people.

Don't bring people problems
Bring them solutions

This mental framework sounds like basic advice but it's linked closely to "Ask not 'can I have' but 'how can I earn?'".

It's a small shift in your thinking from being **expective and reactive** to the world to being **engaging and proactive.** This is most commonly seen in the workforce but you see it at ages as young as two years old. It all boils down to the same habit: we want others to solve our problems so that we don't have to invest the time and thought to do it ourselves. This desire does two things to harm us.

The first is that it weakens us mentally because we're not exercising our own minds in problem solving skills. This is a reason why most legitimate parenting books will advise new parents to let their child struggle to accomplish goals (within reason) such as crawling over pillows or figuring out a puzzle or climbing a tree. Problem solving is a real mental skill that can be developed or, unfortunately for many people, underdeveloped.

The second negative thing our desire to let others fix our problems does is it gives those around us reason to hold us in little regard, to not trust us and to want to be rid of us in some extreme cases. We see people who bring us only problems as a nuisance, an irritant or even a pest. We have a tendency to avoid others by instinct when they begin to act solely as the bringer of bad news. We associate them with negativity and misfortune.

Being able to identify a problem isn't a bad thing. As the old saying goes, identifying the problem is half the battle. But there's a world of difference between those who can **identify the problem** and those who **do something about it.**

Imagine a tornado siren. Most people are annoyed with them even when there is reason to fear a storm. Other than a brief warning slightly before a storm they don't provide much else, not even a sense of safety.

But a tornado shelter? That's much different.

People see a tornado shelter as a godsend and have much more deserved appreciation for the shelter. They invest time and money in a solid tornado shelter and it can give a sense of security they otherwise wouldn't have.
So don't be a tornado siren, at least not exclusively. Be a tornado shelter.

Don't bring people problems, bring solutions.

Be glad you're alive
You have no idea what the
other side is like

Like several of our topics, let's start dark and work our way toward the light.

There's a man named Ken Baldwin who is known for many things from writing to acting to salsa dancing and fishing.

He's also known for one other darker story: at the age of twenty-eight, he chose to end his life.

He drove to the peak of the Golden Gate Bridge, looked out on the bay and jumped from the railing. This story wouldn't be worth telling if it wasn't for two reasons.

The first is that he survived.
The second are his thoughts on the matter.

Once his hands let go of the rail and the possibility of his life ending there became all but guaranteed, Ken had a revelation, "I realized that everything in my life that I thought was unfixable was totally fixable; except for having just jumped."

People tend to mix up when to look at the big picture and when to get lost in the moment. Usually we get it backwards. When times are good, we keep trying to leave the moment and distract ourselves with entertainment, planning, busywork and mindless activity like our phones and streaming services and social media. But when times are tough, we get tunnel vision. We get bogged down in the moment and forget how much more to life there is than our immediate suffering. We forget how precious life is and how little we know of what lies after this one.

There's an old saying that 'the devil you know is better than the devil you don't'. For the most part, this is true. It's easy to get caught up in our troubles. No life is exempt from its own unique pattern of pain. But pain can make us do stupid things, like assume that 'anything is better than this'. Wishful thinking will not end our suffering. But gratitude for every tiny thing that's real about life can take the sting from that suffering away.

Where our focus goes, our vision enhances.
We are living beings and so our focus should be on the joys of *life* however small they may be. It could be the gift of fresh air in your lungs or a full stomach. It could be the last smile someone gave you or the sound of birds you forgot were there until now. You can be grateful for somebody to love or for something small to laugh at. Even our pain can be something to embrace. We can be thankful for the resilience it induced us to have, or the opportunity it opened up that we didn't realize until our advantages were removed.
So when your life darkens exponentially, and the grass on the other side starts looking a little greener remember two things.
The first is that there's so much more to be grateful for in this life if you're only willing to look around and ask for help if you can't.
The second is that you and I (and everyone else that's still above ground) have no idea what exactly is on the other side.

Stick around.

Food is medicine and medicine is food

We live in an over medicated, under exercised, overfed and undernourished society.

Occam's Razor implies that when multiple choices of equal possibility present themselves, the simplest answer, or the one that makes the least amount of assumptions, is the most prudent to trust. When we feel bad many of us prefer to open up the medicine cabinet or go see a doctor to get a prescription or treatment. Every stomachache, migraine, sore back, sleep problem, energy problem, cough and complexion issue seems to have another pill or cream to save us.

I would be willing to bet that many of us could be helped more by adding *less* new things into our body and instead *replacing* gunk with gold.

I'm not here to advocate for the abolition of medicine. What I'm saying is that the pendulum has swung too far in the direction of overmedicating life. In all honesty, most of our problems can be at least alleviated if not cured by what we put into our bodies everyday; our food and drink. Our bodies are incredibly complex biological machines. Introducing a new list of chemicals into our system to fix one problem will never fix that one thing only. Furthermore, you'd be surprised what you see when you turn over the bag of chips at the store and see how much extra stuff is entering your body that *isn't* food.

It's no secret anymore that a huge portion of the food presented to us in restaurants and stores is pure garbage that wasn't actually meant for long term human consumption. We have sacrificed our greater health for the ease and occasional affordability of fast food and processed food (Today, you don't even have the advantage of affordability with fast food). No one ever regrets eating healthier. But millions of people each day regret that bag of potato chips or that sugar syrup concoction at Starbucks or that cheeseburger.

So when we find ourselves facing these health problems, it may be helpful to ask the questions that cost zero dollars:
 "What am I putting in my body that I shouldn't?"
"What can I consume *instead* that could actually help me fight these physical problems?"

You don't need to go to a doctor to eat a banana and get more vitamins. You don't need to spend an extra fifty dollars at CVS for protein when you can enjoy some home cooked chicken and beef. Black coffee can keep you up just as well as Monster and won't leave you twitching from a sugar rush and insulin spike.

You'll live healthier (and keep more of your money) when you realize that food is medicine and medicine is food.

You can only have one priority

"Priorities" is a new word.

Up until quite recently in world languages, there was not a plural form of the word "priority". The word simply came in its singular form and meant the first or 'prior' thing. We all have a thousand things that are important to us. We could fill a page with things to worry about or spend our effort and time on. But a person can't move in more than one direction at a time. You can't dedicate your focus on two things at once.

We've already discussed having a base and setting levels of importance. Building on that premise, you can find your priority through your faith first, then your family then your community.
Your *faith* will tell you how to build your family.
Your *family* will help you determine what community to become a part of.
Your *community* will have needs that can be met by something you have to offer. More often than not, you can find your mission and its priority there. That doesn't mean that you can never have more than one concern. Life is much too layered for that. But everyday you should ask yourself if the one priority or goal of your day was met. If it was, then you're moving in the right direction. Don't get distracted by too many "urgent" matters.

You can only have one priority.

Practice creativity
(art, music, writing, building, etc.)

The mind is a creative force. That much is beyond objection.

We don't just process information from our senses. We order it, interpret it, rearrange it, determine possibilities and potential. We all have a method of expressing creativity whether we think of ourselves as an "artist" or "musician" or not.

Some of us are gifted in more traditional methods of creativity like painting, drawing, playing an instrument, singing or writing (For your sake, I sincerely hope I have skill in the latter).

But many of us carry creative power in other ways we didn't think of as 'creative'. We create landscapes for our yards, collect soldiers to construct historical war scenes, and design our homes to be beautiful and open spaces. We build incredible spreadsheets that take chaos of information and bring order and sense to it. We create conversation filled with levity and joy amongst friends by having a sharp sense of humor. Anytime you have taken material from the outside world and changed it based on an idea in your mind, you have successfully expressed creativity.

We're built to create. A healthy mind is one that doesn't just *process* but *contributes* to reality. What also benefits your mind is learning something new. A great habit to continue growing in life is to pick one creative endeavor and practice it until you see significant improvement.

Building competence builds more than just confidence. It builds networks in your mind that connect to a billion other areas of thinking. Learning to play the trumpet may not seem to help you in your job at the bank or in your high school precalculus class. But your brain is finding new ways to interpret problems, determine patterns and meaning and find solutions. It may not help your football skills to learn to paint at first glance but learning to see things differently and find visual opportunities can be a bigger help than you realize. Our communities are a better place when we're creating and growing. It's one area we can always do so, even in old age.

So never stop growing and practice creativity.

The devil is in the details

"I have read the terms and conditions"

You read this line and click the box and sign up for whatever it is you were interested in. It's the one lie everyone seems to make.
This isn't an internet safety talk. This is a piece of advice and a mental framework for you to **pay attention!**

More often than not, a slight miscalculation or a small overlooked detail is the problem that crumbles an operation, a business, an army or a relationship. Entire court cases are made based on interpretation of one word or phrase. Military strategy depends on the smallest bits of data from wind direction to the amount of doors in a given building. A life can be permanently changed based on a number on a license plate, the penny miscounted on taxes, a quote given out of context or remembering an anniversary date.

Politicians use this to their advantage. Data is a slippery practice and minds can easily be changed based on how a 'public servant' in a slick suit frames a piece of information. What they show you is almost *always* a small fraction of the information you need to know to understand the full story.

Reading the fine print is more than just double checking your document when buying a car or signing up for a subscription. It's also the practice of thinking critically and logically about the meaning of what you are being told. It can be challenging and boring at times. It's easier to take everything at face value especially for young men who tend to look at life in broad ideas rather than minute details. But the advantages of going through life with your eyes open are countless. Like a sprained ankle, it's almost never going to be the large obstacle that trips you up. It's certainly going to be a small hole or bump.

To stay safe remember, the devil is in the details.

Freedom and security
are mutually exclusive

If you've never read the Bible or even parts of it, I would highly recommend it; even those who are not Christian or Jewish. In the book of Exodus, the Israelites are slaves in Egypt. After Moses communes with God he is told to free the Isrealites from Pharaoh. Through Moses, God works miracles and plagues upon the Egyptian people until Pharoah relents to freeing the Israelites and sending them off into the desert.

Here's where it gets interesting.

The Jewish people had been begging and crying out to God for freedom. They had been beaten and scorched in the Egyptian heat, toiling away as slaves and suffering each and every day. Now, by the hand of God, they were free to enter the world and make their own fate. With the protection of the highest power in the universe, they could roam across the desert to find the promised land that they were destined to enjoy.

But after only a few days of freedom, they began to complain. They sulked and groaned to Moses that they would die of starvation out in the desert and that it was better to be slaves in Egypt because at least they had food and a house to sleep in. Any sane person feels a bit of incredulity when reading that. We can't imagine not wanting freedom, especially here in America. But if you think deeper, it's pretty reflective of human nature.

Most people don't really want freedom. We want security. We cannot have both because every step towards security is a step away from our own care for ourselves and into someone else's care and authority. Freedom means we inherit all the *choices* and also the *consequences* of those choices; the good, the bad and the ugly.

So many of us look at the two opposites and pick security. We want to be taken care of and we want to know where our bed is and when our next meal is. Freedom carries risk. It means that you're extending yourself and living on your own labor and success. It can be frightening. But what's important to keep in mind is that suffering and risk will happen whether we have security *or* freedom. The only difference is that when you choose freedom, you choose your suffering and how to respond to it. When you choose security, your suffering will come at the hand of someone else in one form or another. Even the slaves had the security of food and shelter. So do cows before the slaughter.

So when you go about life and pick your career or your community or cast your vote, remember that freedom and security are mutually exclusive.

Choose wisely.

If the product is "free"
you're the product

This is a new problem in the world.

Other than slavery and serfdom, there has never been an area of life where people themselves are the product of human interest and commerce. But today, you cannot escape the eyes and interest of corporations, government entities, scammers, pirates and political pundits. Everybody wants a piece of you for their spreadsheet, database, survey, sales list, banking info, debt info or myriad other items.

So when you see that an account or a membership or loans or anything else has the "free" label on it, be skeptical.
Nothing is free in life; everything carries a cost. It's not always money. Sometimes it's time, effort, patience, safety or even...you. Your credit card number may not be going into the boxes on your screen but you're putting *something* in and that something has value to someone.

The best takeaway from this mental framework is to understand the product that's actually being sold and the actual cost that's being asked for it. That doesn't mean you can't trust people or you need to treat everyone like a sleazy salesman. It does mean to be observant of that four letter word and all the hidden context around it.
 Sunsets are free. Social media accounts? Not so much. They may not charge you money for having an account but they're taking something from you.

Believe it.

What is *important* is not always what is *urgent*

One of the hardest things about adult life is that there are no shortage of concerns that pry at our attention. Compounding this issue is the fact that with the dawn of cell phones and later smartphones and WiFi, every matter that concerns us can now have full access to us anytime, anywhere regardless of how we try to manage our time.

Let's look at Haley's day.

Today's box in her planner includes paying the power bill, walking and feeding her dog, filling the car up with gas, getting the groceries, turning in that project report to her boss, moving the trash to the curb, dropping some checks off at the bank, signing up for the seminar she had planned to get more assertiveness skills and getting her hair cut, showered up and ready before her date tonight at seven thirty.

It can feel overwhelming and it's no surprise that in the feeble mental state of many adults in the modern world, some people find it hard to even get out of bed when looking at their planner. One thing that can do a tremendous amount of good is recognizing that something that is **important** to do is not always an **urgent** thing that needs to get done *right now*.

Let's look back at the example of Haley's busy day.

Her date is important to her. So is the seminar and getting signed up for it. The stylist will be open all day and she still has a quarter of a tank of gas to get through the day with. Her house is also only two minutes away from the bank and she can always use the ATM if the building itself is closed. So out of her list of important things to do, what is *urgent* for her?

She has a dog, a living being, that she has to take care of. So she starts the day with feeding and walking her dog. She takes the garbage out next because the trash men usually come at nine in the morning so the time crunch requires her to handle it early. From there she goes to work where she can finish up her report to submit by noon and on her lunch break she tackles the sign up and payment to go to her seminar next month. She also pays her power bill during her break and after work, she fills up on gas and gets her hair cut.
Before coming home she stops and picks up the week's groceries from the store and arrives home by six fifteen with enough time to put the groceries away and get ready to be picked up at seven thirty.

Haley took her entire list of important things to do that day and structured her day around what was most necessary to do quickly, what was urgent, and handled it first. Then she went through the list and tackled other important things that did not have as strict of a timeline around them.

This is a highly important skill to function in the world. Whenever you feel stressed out about your day it can help tremendously to make a list of your day's activities and the timeline that it needs to be done by and how much time it will take to do it. From there you can separate what is unimportant, what is important and what is urgent.

Learn the difference.

Think first of your responsibilities
then about your rights

The bottom line is, rights are an outgrowth of responsibilities. You are born with a purpose and your rights also have a purpose which is giving you the freedom to fulfill your responsibilities. The right to vote is worthless if you don't fulfill your responsibility of being a contributing and knowledgeable citizen. Your right to free speech means very little if you have nothing worthwhile to say because you're not responsible with your words. Your right to life is forfeit if you ignore your responsibility to other people's lives and endanger them.

With all the stress lately over everybody's rights, it's helpful to ask the people demanding them what their actual *duties* are. Many times our duties will outline where our rights actually lie, not the other way around.

If you're a student in school, ask yourself first what you're responsible for. It's to learn as much truth as possible to become a well formed and prepared adult. That will point you to where your rights are.
You have the right to be told the truth, to be provided a proper knowledge designed to prepare you to be a successful and contributing citizen. You have the right to be challenged and face adversity to make you tough against the opposition you'll face in the world.

If you are a low wage worker, your responsibility is to learn as much as possible, earning skills and conducting yourself in a manner that helps the business succeed and gives you the resume boost to rise to a better position with more pay and benefits.

That means you have the right to know what job you are supposed to be doing, be instructed efficiently on how to do it correctly and be given the tools and resources to execute the job including the agreed upon price and terms of your hiring. If either you or your employer breaks the agreement, either of you has the right to walk away.

So take control of your life and evaluate what your duties are and then you can fulfill them by ensuring those correlative rights allow you to do so.

Working smart and hard are not mutually exclusive
Do them both

You've most likely heard both cliches to always 'be the hardest worker in the room' and also to 'work smart, not hard'.

Why not both?

There's a time to plot your path and choose the most prudent way to go about a task to reduce unnecessary effort. There's also a time to shut up, put your head down and do the required grunt work to get a hard job done. As a general rule of thumb, working smart comes first chronologically. Determine what needs to be done, how to go about it and what and who you need to fulfill the task. Next comes the inevitable hard work.

You'll need both qualities to truly succeed in life but if I had to bias one over the other at a young age, you can survive the longest on working hard in this world. The long history of humanity has proven that. As the old saying goes, "hard work beats talent when talent doesn't work hard". The younger you are, the more important it is to know the value of hard work. Time will give you the wisdom of experience to refine your skills and knowledge to find the best and most efficient ways to do things. But if you never learn to push yourself through the worst parts of a job, then all the 'smart work' in the world won't save you.

So work hard **and** work smart.

Don't be ashamed of privilege
Be ashamed of wasting it

A common insult I've seen bandied about today is that a person is 'privileged'.

It's a phrase that's been used with different subcategories depending on the recipient of the charge. I've heard of 'white privilege', 'male privilege', 'wealth privilege' and other more obscure versions.

I won't address the merits of the charge since in my opinion I believe we are *all* privileged far beyond our ability to deny. From the most fortunate to the most destitute of us all, we are given a chance at salvation by God to enter Heaven after death. I consider that privilege enough.

But assuming that it is true that people can be privileged in a variety of ways such as wealth or status, I don't consider privilege to be an inherently bad thing. We are *all* born with gifts and advantages given to us by God. It would be no better for us to be ashamed of our families wealth or connections than it would be for a lizard to be ashamed of his tail or a dog her canine teeth. We are given what we are given. Simple as that.

What we should be ashamed of is *wasting* the gifts and advantages God gives us through our families by denying them, rejecting them or using them for evil. With every privilege we receive, we should show gratitude by actively using it for the good of God, the good of our family and the good of our community.

Don't be ashamed of privilege. Be ashamed of wasting it.

Ask questions, be curious and skeptical

Children have a unique ability to learn quicker than any other stage of human development. Older generations have a better ability to sniff out bull crap than any other age group.
The trick in life is making the most of both of these two skills.

Curiosity and skepticism work like two opposite senses, complimenting each other and giving you a bigger, more defined picture of reality.

Curiosity gives you the drive to learn more and gain knowledge while skepticism gives you the instinct to think critically about what you're finding out to either dispose of it and forget it or hang on to it for use in the future. You'll find extraordinary examples of both in society.
Men like Leonardo da Vinci, Albert Einstein and Mike Rowe had/have a profound sense of wonder and a passion to find out more about the world and all that's in it. What was important to them was the desire to know how things work, what they're made out of and detect patterns across the universe. Their work and others like them, has defined the course of human progress for thousands of years.
 They are the spearheads of humanity.

Men like Thomas Sowell, Winston Churchill, Thomas Jefferson and Socrates are known for a different reason. The main trait that these men shared contributes to our clarity of thought and through them, we have understood the world better because of their harsh criticism of bad ideas, sloppy thinking and false ideology. Thousands of terrible notions have been discarded on the ash heap of history and it is men like these who have helped to put them there before the damage those notions could inflict destroyed civilization.

We need both of these gifts from people amongst us. We can do wonders for our world by sharpening these gifts within ourselves. Cultivate both of them by asking questions.

Be curious and be skeptical.

Your leaders
are *not*
your friends

We all want to have friends in high places. Getting cool connections with people, whether it's the CEO of a large company, the police chief or the local congressman, it can be an exciting experience being friends with someone who can get you into places that you wouldn't be otherwise.

But when the person is *your* leader, *your* CEO, *your* congressman, things change. Part of being a good leader is being able to make decisions apart from personal feelings, preferences or connections. The role of a leader, a good one anyway, is to work for the betterment of an entire group without fear or favor from one segment of the population.

This quality in a person comes with a tough demand; separation from the group.
That isn't to say that a good leader has nothing in common with those who follow him or is unwilling to have some candid moments with those she leads but a true leader has necessary space between themselves and those they have authority over.

Being a leader may require a boss to give a promotion to someone he doesn't like or a mother to correct her child for staying out too late. It may require a teacher to hold his student accountable or a congresswoman to choose a policy that causes her social group to cut her off from the fancy parties because it's the best choice for her constituents.

Being a friend to those you lead, including as a parent, only compromises your ability to lead or be led properly. It adds a layer of unnecessary consideration to any decision and can add misery to choices that need to be made but are not popular. Friendships are, by definition, relationships based on closeness. Leadership is a relationship that requires some distance.

That distance is a safety barrier against personal animus or advantage of one over another. A team, a company, or a nation will operate better if you do *not* select your leaders based on who you are friends with or could 'sit down and have a beer with'. This is a dangerous recipe that creates shallow standards for leadership.

If you want to be a part of anything worthwhile remember that your leaders are *not* your friends.

Respect your elders
They've seen your world
and the one before it

Age is a beautiful thing.

I know, I know, the whole world screams in anguish at the mere mention of age. Women squirm when you ask them their age. Men over forty will bristle and puff out their chest as if to show that their old glory days are not yet over. Half of the ads online push creams and fillers and pills and diets and tanners and clothing all with the purpose of hiding age and pretending it doesn't exist. We live in a society that says "age is just a number" and makes every effort to convince people of it.

This is a new phenomenon. Previous generations understood that old age was a badge of honor. It means you have a much deeper and richer experience of life. It means that you have a wealth of wisdom that can only come from time and a life well lived. It meant that you were a survivor; that you had been through the fires of life and lived to tell the tale. People would look to their elders for advice and leadership instead of Hollywood airheads and talented yet shallow musicians and athletes.

That respect for grandma and grandpa was hard earned. They had lived every year of a young person's life and then done it again twofold. They've walked every step of life from childhood to angsty teenager to struggling adult, to starting a family, to raising a home full of children to working through long careers and making it successfully to retirement. For them, it is like having lived in multiple worlds or having played at higher levels than us 'youngsters'. They've seen cultures come and go. They've seen fashion fads rise and fade. They've seen all that has changed in their many years of life and most important of all, they have seen what has NOT changed like human nature and morality and objective truth.

Talking to your grandparents can give you more wisdom for your road ahead than any YouTube influencer, news anchor or celebrity crush you have.

So when it comes to who should get the lion's share of your respect, look to your elders.

They've seen your world and the one before it.

Confidence is cultivated through repetitions of success

Confidence and **bluster** look similar at first glance but stand a world apart.

Bluster is a fool's arrogance; a feeling of strength based on nothing but delusion or wishful thinking. A kid who's never stepped on a skateboard in his life hops on it with bluster, thinking he'll glide effortlessly along the concrete. His bluster is based on ignorance of his own lack of skill and delusion from seeing experts do so after years of practice. He jumps on...and eats cement. He may get up with less teeth than he went down with.

Confidence is what happens when you trust the process of hard work, focus and consistency and know that over time, the formula will in fact succeed. Everyone can improve at anything by that same formula.

Now point this mental framework at yourself: what do *you* lack confidence in?
Driving a car?
Calculus?
Getting that girl you like to go on a date with you?
Whatever it is, if you follow the line of thinking from the paragraph above, you'll realize how to gain that desired confidence.
You need to focus on what skill must be learned and how to do it. Then you need to practice it with consistency and determination.

Get in the car with your dad and dedicate an entire week on highway merging and parallel parking. Do it over and over again until not only does the task no longer intimidate you, but it seems boring and repetitive.

Sit down with a tutor everyday and work through those formulas one by one with practice problems until you understand them forwards and backwards.

Talk to the girls around you everyday regardless of your initial awkwardness, having respectful conversations until you are just as comfortable talking to them as your own friends. Tell jokes, ask questions, listen to answers, tell stories and share insights. Talk with them so much that they become the first people you walk in a room to speak with.

Your confidence will build as your skills do because they are based on repetitions of success.

Separate the man from the message

One unfortunate mindset that plagues us and has done so with increasing intensity is the 'halo effect'.

The **halo effect** is a process of thinking in which we assume that the positive traits of a person or thing must transfer to other areas of life. For instance, we may look at an advertisement with our favorite baseball player enjoying a sports drink. We see him take a swig of it on TV and unconsciously assume that because he's a great baseball player, he must also be a great source on the price, flavor and effectiveness of that sports drink.

We look at Hollywood celebrities and make the same mistake of believing that because they are great actresses and actors who are attractive, they must also be experts on political candidates, social concerns and global conflict.

But the person is not the same as the message.

Believing information based solely on the person delivering it can cause you to vote for the wrong candidate, choose the wrong job, abandon your faith or cause myriad other harms in your life.

This trend also works in reverse. We see a man who's earned negative headlines for a personal foible and so we choose to ignore his opinions on matters that he specializes in or has proven himself to be correct on before. What applies on the positive is true for the negative. If you want to make the most educated decisions, judge the information on its *own* merits.

You are the average of the five people you spend the most time around
Choose wisely

This is an oldie but a goodie.

If I may make one adaptation, I will do so at the very end. There's a reason why our parents have so much of an influence on us. We spend a vast majority of our early lives with them and around them. Each of us is an individual capable of making our own choices counter to what outside influences are doing. However, we are also creatures of inertia meaning we pick the path of least resistance or habit more often than not. When it comes to our behavior and habits, we mimic what those closest to us are doing whenever we're in doubt or not strongly opinionated about a certain thing. This is especially true for people we admire and look up to. Our social impulse demands this and so we tailor our general habits from what we see each day. This is something to be conscious of when you start making friends and associates. There's nothing wrong with having lots of friends and acquaintances.

But ask yourself what kind of people do you spend the most time with? Do they make you better? Do they inspire you to be more than what you are or do you find yourself stooping to worse behavior in their presence?

My one dispute with the general phrase is that it assumes your influences are the normal people around you. Earlier I mentioned the importance of placing God first and foremost in your life.
 Let's be clear: God is real. He's also perfect. With perfection as your rubric and if you spend the plurality of

your time in prayer or consciousness of your divine creator, imagine how impactful that will be on your character.

As a Catholic, we believe in sitting in the physical presence of God through adoration. During this time, the bread that has been blessed and has become the Body of Christ or the Eucharist, is placed in a holy monstrance in the chapel or church and set on an altar. People can come in and sit quietly in peace with the Lord. Most come to sit without ever speaking a word. I've done it myself. I'd highly recommend it. It gives you a profound sense of peace, especially during turbulent times in your life.

So, with that being said, if you make yourself the average of the one *divine* being and the four *other* quality people you spend the most time with, you'll be set up quite well in life.

Be professional not just in your career endeavors, but also in your personal life

You'd be amazed at how much you can do with so little effort.

This mental framework is a key example of that. If you make a small point to dress and behave as if your future employers and colleagues are around you, your conduct will be high and above the vast majority of people in society. I wish this wasn't true but it most certainly is today.

If you'd like an example, look up from whatever public place you may be in right now or going to. How many people are dressed in pajamas or wearing flip flops in a restaurant? How many adults are sitting next to their family or friends but ignoring them by staring at their phone? How many employees have you seen behind a register cursing and laughing with their friends instead of providing the service they're paid to provide? How many people are slouching in chairs, slurring their words or have hair that looks like it was styled with a weed eater? How many people at the grocery store are showing more skin than you'd see at a beach?

These are all things that scream one thing: a lack of professionalism. And the more important of a job they have, the more terrifying it is to see that trait. It's one thing to see your barista act a little careless with your coffee like he just woke up three minutes before you arrived. It's another thing to see your pilot or surgeon in the hospital lobby act the same way or go on a screaming tirade on X or do ridiculous TikTok dances.

Professionalism is an unhailed quality today and those who can display it always shine brighter than those who don't. It requires discipline, forethought and consistency. It can earn you respect, opportunity and more legitimate connections and relationships in life. It tells others that you have more to offer than what your transcript or resume or test scores provide. And it's contagious to other areas of your life and to the people you spend time with. Everyone is made better from a professional demeanor.

So be professional.

Everywhere.

All the time.

You always need to have these five connections:
Doctor, Lawyer, Banker, Real Estate Agent, Cop

This list has been made and remade a million different ways by a million different people. The general point is the same:

You can't do it all on your own, so build real relationships with people of a *variety* of skills and knowledge. Don't just stick with your work friends or college buddies. There are certain areas of life where understanding can be the difference between financial, medical or legal detriment and success. Making a point to have friends in your circle who you can go to for advice and counsel can save you a lot of grief from time to time.

Sometimes it can be hard to trust a mechanic not to screw you on the bill or a doctor to give you a straight answer on the diagnosis. Experts can lie just as easily as anybody so it can help to have friends in different fields who you already have a built trust in to ask honest questions and get honest answers. Not to mention, your friends will be more likely to answer that panicked call at three in the morning than the guy just clocking in and clocking out of work.

Connections provide a trusted and diverse sense of community in your life. The best way to establish these connections is through your church, community and work. Meet people, be professional and show charity, grace and wit as often as you can. Connections will come along the way. It pairs quite nicely with the previous mental framework. Just be sure not to seek these connections out for their own sake. People aren't products on a checklist so if you think of your friends and realize you don't know any good lawyers, don't go searching online under 'Legal Help' for a drinking buddy. Let these friends come about naturally just like any others.

Show virtue in your ways all the time and the people you need will come on God's schedule.

Health is wealth

Quality of life is just as important as longevity.

We admire the Lamborghini going down the highway or the yacht at the harbor, not realizing that the heavyset man in each one still wheezes to put on his socks or has to take blood pressure pills from terrible lifestyle habits. *Wealth comes in more forms than just money.* One of them is our physical strength and vitality. We all lose it over time. But maintaining our peak performance for as long as possible can be the difference between enjoying another year of life and dreading it. At twenty years old, most young men and women are "in the grind" trying to earn as much money as quickly as possible. That can lead to some dreadful eating and exercise habits from staying late at work, eating out and sitting at a desk for decades in a row. Some people do make a point to stay in shape but many get into bad eating and activity habits while relying on their youthful metabolism to keep them trim.

But life hits you fast.

Our metabolism slows down. We get aches and pains. We get sick. We slow down. We break down. Remember that while you are earning and rising in income, you want a good life to actually enjoy it. Take time to take care of your physical, mental and spiritual health. These are precious forms of wealth too easily overlooked in search of the "almighty dollar". All the money in the world won't help you if you're tearing your life up in other ways.

Health is wealth.

You will not be judged by your mistakes, but by your ability to fix your mistakes speedily and the discipline to not repeat them

Some mistakes go down in history.

Japan bombing Pearl Harbor.
Napoleon at Waterloo.
The Red Sox trading Babe Ruth.

Some people live on in history as embarrassing failures because of mistakes they made. You have to feel bad for the guy who just played the wrong hand in the history books. But for the vast majority of people, we are known by those around us for our ability to learn from our inevitable mistakes and turn each one into a personal guide for how to improve.

Except for the most impatient and graceless of people, everyone understands that we all make mistakes. We forget to send that document. We oversleep or forget our lunch. We zig when we should've zagged or zag when we should've zigged. Must of us shrug our shoulders when that person 'steps in it'. But what makes a friend, coworker or spouse so aggravating to be around is the mistakes that happen *consistently* and without any indication of *change*.

Imagine a car that always failed to start in the morning for work. No matter how many times you brought it into a shop and sank money into it, it would fail every morning. It would drive you crazy. You'd start shopping for a new one after a week. There's only so much time and energy we can spend on repetitive failure. It's important to not be that car in people's lives. Don't fail the same way at the same thing over and over again without making adjustments.

Show some awareness and discipline by figuring out what you did wrong, making the conscious decision to do something else to avoid that mistake and then committing to the change.

That's what the world will judge you by.

Learn the language of money

There are a multitude of statistics that show how the average American is struggling more and more to handle inflation, debt, housing and more. Retirement plans have never been more scarcely thought out and the age of retirement has been pushed further and further back.

Understanding the flow of money is a bit of a science mixed with art. Knowing how to make money work *for* you instead of the other way around is a skill that is expressed by too few but can be learned by just about anyone with the desire and determination to do so. As long as money is not the end game for your ambition, learning the language of money can be a tool to improve your life and more importantly, the lives of those around you. Like any other skill, it can be put to incorrect use but the ability to direct the flow of money efficiently in your life isn't inherently bad and can save you a lot of headaches in your adult life. This is especially important when you consider the fact that many businesses and government officials who would take your money would put it to uses that you find immoral and possibly evil.

When you begin with your mission to learn this new language, be sure to take your knowledge from those who have established a long history of success over time, not internet gurus, quick success stories or social media 'flexers'. Anyone, even those with no understanding of money, can earn a quick fortune based on circumstance or skill in a trade or service. But not everyone has shown time-tested wealth maintenance and growth. Do your research on who to listen to.

Learn the language of money.

Become process oriented

I will repeat that material wealth is *not* the end all, be all of existence but it's intriguing to note that all of the most recurring millionaire professions are process oriented jobs : Engineers, Accountants, Teachers, Business Executives, and Attorneys.
'Teachers' may sound unbelievable but when you think of how broad that term is, it's not a far-fetched idea.

So what is being "process oriented"?

This is a term that means to clearly define goals based on a desire or need to fix a problem, setting specific chronological steps to get there and single mindedly attacking each step until its completion.

Most people fail at some area of this system. We fail to recognize a problem or can't define our desire or goal. When we get those right we struggle to break down the steps to get there and even if we get that far, we unravel quickly due to lack of focus or trying to attack two steps at a time. It's difficult to do so but if it is managed, even for the slightest of tasks, it pays dividends in the amount of ground you can cover in any area of life.

If you feel intimidated by a major project, start off small. Like any skill you'll need a little skill building and ramping up. Practice setting up small and relatively easy goals, writing down the steps to get there and knocking out each step systematically. You can do this for job applications, cleaning your bathroom or doing your lawn work. You'll improve over time at this.

Become process oriented.

Invest in the future

There are three main things that will outlive you in a positive way and will continue to give to others long after you're gone.

Planting a tree.
Writing a book.
Having children.

Not everyone may be called to fulfill every one of these tasks but the general point is to go through this life with a determination to give regardless of whether you will see the full fruits of your labor.

Planting a tree displays gratitude for your home, for the life you have been given and the world around you. It shows trust in those that come after you; that they will have the same appreciation for life to keep that tree alive and to one day enjoy its cool shade, the sound of wind through its leaves or the sight of living creatures that will reside in it in years to come.

Writing a book tells the world that you believe in something strongly, you have the confidence to proclaim it and the determination to see the vision in your head become a real and tangible thing that people can hold in their hands. Any moron can blather a quick line on social media but to sit down and carefully construct your story or your message can be a monumental task. The most extraordinary feeling, though, is when you go through that entire process and realize through your readers that someone else out there shares your same vision. I did not have nearly enough respect for authors until I tried to accomplish this task.

Having children has already been a topic of discussion earlier in this book but it is worth touching up on once more. A vast majority of men and women are called to have children. Of the three investments in the future, this one shows the greatest faith and love. It is in this venture that you will endure more pain, strife, anxiety, heartache and frustration. But with these crosses that you *willingly* bear, you will experience more love, joy, excitement, nostalgia, warmth, fulfillment, carefree timelessness and purpose than you could ever imagine in a life lived without children. It is my firm belief that a sinister mark of our time is the amount of leaders we have in this world with no children. That shows a lack of faith or investment in the future of the nations they lead.

The world is made more beautiful by the care each generation puts into the ones that follow. It flourishes with each investment made in which the investor expects no personal return on it. We're made better when our predecessors 'pay it forward' and we have the chance to give these same gifts to the ones who follow us.

Invest in the future.

Not making a decision
is a still a decision

Indecision is a common quality in our population today. It plagues every relationship, every business, every social interaction.
Where should we eat?
What should I do after graduation?
Where should I work?
What do I do about that leak?
The answer to all of these questions should not be 'I don't know'. At least, not for very long.
The temptation to kick the can down the road is a normal impulse and it means the same thing universally: We don't want the consequences of committing to an action. Once we decide to do something we either fail or succeed in doing it. We accept the costs and risks of whatever results in our decision. But remember this: Time flies regardless of whether you pick a given choice or not. Your life ticks away whether you pick a road or a road is picked for you. The truth of the matter is, even if someone else chooses for you, you still decided to have them do so.
You still made a decision.
Your life is better lived when you take full command of it by making a real decision and not pawning off the results of your life to another flawed human being. Everyone has enough problems handling their own life. Don't put your life and it's decision making on to them as well.

Be decisive.

If you genuinely try your best, you **cannot** lose.

This sounds like either a bold claim by a coach or a reassuring comment made by mom after you lost a soccer game...but it's true.

For one thing, it's actually incredibly hard to fail at something after a long period of single minded effort. There is no skill you cannot make incredible progress in with enough time and focus. So the chances of you failing after truly and honestly trying your hardest are actually smaller than you think.

Nonetheless, even if you do technically fail at the task you are attempting after full throttle effort, you still didn't lose. You gained *something* from that effort. You grew in more ways than you can fully appreciate until days, weeks and sometimes years later. Sometimes the areas of victory are hard to see like the mental and emotional growth that can stem from devoted effort.

Other times, your failure after trying can give you skills and experience that prove useful in other endeavors. As the saying goes, when one door closes, a window opens. The greatest men and women in the world failed thousands of times...but they didn't necessarily lose. So be patient with yourself and make the clear decision to do everything to your greatest ability.

If you do that, you just can't lose.

Avoid temptation

There's a line Catholics say during Confession that I have always liked. After we confess our sins, we recite what is called the **Act of Contrition** in which we humbly express our sorrow for our sins and resolve to not sin again.
I know, I know, we all end up *right* back in that confessional for more sins and usually, they are the same ones. But the point of the prayer is not that we expect to be perfect from now on but to express our determination to try and try again.
The Lord ponders the heart after all.
The reason I bring this up is because there is a specific phrase that I gravitate towards and think about often :
"I firmly intend, with Your help,to do penance, to sin no more, **and to avoid whatever leads me to sin.**"
Did you catch it?
I mean, I put it in bold so I'm guessing you did. We don't just pray to not sin. We also get to the *root* of the problem and vow to avoid even putting ourselves in the same situation that is conducive to that sin.
This is probably the most neglected part of every Catholic's life. We promise to sin no more but we completely overlook avoiding the people, places and things that make it so easy for us to sin that way in the first place.
But the problem is much more common than just in the Catholic church. Everybody sins and screws up. And everybody places themselves in situations they know are not helping them in life.
One key to avoiding the same damned mistakes over and over again is breaking out of the cycle by avoiding the starting point of it in the first place.

Alcoholics participating in AA are constantly in a state of remembering this piece of advice. They avoid bars and social situations in which alcohol is everywhere. Participants of Narcotics Anonymous will avoid 'old haunts' and buddies who contributed to their drug habits. But you don't have to be an 'addict' to use this tool.

Do you find yourself overeating at night and making yourself sick? Find ways of avoiding those midnight trips to the fridge. Brush your teeth early. Don't keep sweets in the house or keep them at a friend or neighbor's house. Make it highly inconvenient to follow through on grabbing that bag of Doritos at midnight.

Do you find yourself grabbing your phone and looking up a bunch of crap you shouldn't or 'doom scrolling' with the door locked? Keep your phone charging in another room. Take the lock off your door. Don't take your phone with you to the bathroom.

Do your friends constantly pull you into useless gossip that makes you feel guilty afterwards? Maybe find a new group to spend your lunches with or pick up an activity that doesn't leave you the time to waste on pointless discussions like that.

Father Mike Schmitz has a great quote that hits a similar topic. He says, "Choose the easy 'No', instead of the hard 'No'".

The example is a young couple who chooses to take a romantic night drive and park in a remote place. During that time, things go a little too far and they both feel unready and guilty for having done it.

Which 'No' do you think would have been easier to say:

The 'No' to going on a late night drive alone or

The "No' to engaging in intimacy after the situation has already been set up perfectly to enjoy it?

Take the easy 'No'.

Avoid whatever leads you to sin.

You will lose

That feels like a rude turnaround from earlier, doesn't it?

But yes,
there will be times when you lose; times when you are
supposed to lose. This has nothing to do with trying and
failing and everything to do with the unpredictability of
life. Despite your most fervent prayers and greatest
efforts, things will be taken from you. You don't have
control over that. People who have trouble with this
concept become violently disrupted in their spirit when
this inevitably happens to them. You will lose jobs,
opportunities, relationships and loved ones. The older you
get, the faster you'll lose them, too.

Loss is just as important a part of life as victory. What
transcends any loss in life is where your priorities lie. Your
character and what you give to others will live far beyond
your losses, even your very life. To lose something or
someone does not remove the good that was already done
in your life by what was taken. The friend you said
goodbye to or the mother you had to lay to rest may be
gone, but the value they brought into your life still exists
and can even be passed on to others around you, if you are
resolute enough to do so.

Remember that God is good, in every walk of life, in good
times and in bad;
when you win
and more importantly,
when you lose.

Habits and Tips for a Healthy Life

These tips for living a much more successful and healthy life are ones that I either personally use, have friends who have used or have been passed down in written or spoken advice by some of the most successful people to ever live. They don't require that much explanation and when they do, I will make those explanations as brief as possible.

Try one.

Try some.

Try them all.

Just don't try '*none*'.

Breathe right

Don't be a mouth breather or a shallow breather. Get
proper air into your lungs and brain for better energy,
focus and mental capacity.
Good breathing requires deep, controlled breaths through
your nose.
Some military personnel use what is called 'box
breathing' : Four seconds inhale through the nose, hold
the breath for four seconds, exhale the breath for four
seconds, wait four seconds before drawing in your next
four second breath.
This is a great way to reduce stress and can even help you
sleep in some cases.
When running, breathing right can help you maximize
your energy. Breathe in for three steps and breathe out for
three steps.
A lot can be accomplished if you just breathe right.

Use proper posture

Much of your back pain, neck pain and even hip and knee
pain can be avoided by walking and sitting upright with
your back straight, your chin level and your shoulders
squared.
Don't slouch by letting your neck slink out.
You're not a dinosaur.
It looks bad and over time, it'll make you feel bad.
Use proper posture.

Bathe

Don't be gross.

Brush your teeth twice a day for two minutes
And floss

Same thing. Don't be gross.
Also, you'll save yourself from a *ton* of health problems
and medical bills by keeping your mouth healthy.
Trust me.

Hydrate before bed and as soon as you wake up

This will help you sleep easier, wake up easier and reduce bad breath.

Workout fifteen minutes a day

You don't need that much to keep in shape. Fifteen minutes a day, every day on a consistent level will maintain good physical health for a vast majority of people.
Calisthenics, plyometrics, weight lifting, cross fit, cycling, rock climbing; it doesn't matter. Get your heart rate up for fifteen solid minutes and it will go a very long way for you.

Read fifteen minutes a day

Read the explanation of the previous page and the same applies on a *mental* level for reading. My one precaution is to treat reading like food. Don't read junk food. No 'Fifty Shades of Grey', 'Twilight' or the latest politician's bloviating autobiography. Read books that are edifying, intellectually stimulating and that help you refine your thinking through a pursuit of truth.
Read fifteen minutes a day.

Kill screen time after 9:00 p.m.

If you're under the age of eighteen I would even go so far as to advise you to kill it sooner than that. Your brain doesn't fully develop until the age of twenty-five and blue light, internet access and social media use have proven track records of harming brain development and mental/emotional health.
But if all else fails, by killing all phone, computer, game system and television use after 9:00pm, you will sleep better, have more energy, have more time and be verifiably happier.
If you're looking for something to do with all this new time when you're stuck in line or right before bed, go back to the previous page and read it again.

Look everyone in the eye when speaking

Don't be shifty.
Look me in the eye.

Dress sharp but never flashy

There's a fine line between looking professional and looking like a degenerate at the Met Gala.

Repeat someone's name when you meet them

This is especially important if you suck at remembering names (like me).
If you read *How to Win Friends and Influence People* by Dale Carnegie, you'll know that a huge portion of success in society and the business world will come from remembering people's names.
It's important to them.

Start your day with fruit and protein

Nothing against a good stack of pancakes or french toast
every now and then but fuel your body right when you
start your day. At least get your day off to a running start
with good food before looking at the sugar bombs.
Eat a breakfast of champions.

End your day by writing about it

By writing about your day you will improve your thinking, increase overall recollection, and improve handwriting. Finally, at the end of any given year of doing this, you will see the development of your own life and thinking over time. It's a long game practice, but it's worth it. End your day by writing about it.

Arrive early everywhere you go

If you're early, you're on time.
If you're on time, you're late.
If you're late, that's unacceptable.

Be the first one ready

If you're too young to drive or you don't have your vehicle you may not always be in charge of when you get somewhere. If that's the case, don't be the reason y'all are late.

Add ten percent to your travel time for traffic

or twenty.

Be quick to show positive reactions, slow to show negative ones

A good rule of thumb is to consciously pause for at least a minute when hearing bad news. When you hear good news, let your first reaction shine immediately. Even if you're not a positive person by nature, this practice will give people a much better impression of you.

Three times to put your phone away:
1. At the dinner table
2. At church or a church function
3. When someone is speaking with you

**Have one meal with your family everyday
No excuses**

Say 'Sir' and 'Ma'am' to all adults, no matter what

Start with your parents if you haven't already. You should expect the same when you become an adult. Respect starts small and it goes a long way.

Don't vote just because you're eighteen

Get a job, take some responsibility for someone other than yourself, get educated on the issues at hand and *then* vote. Get some skin in the game *before* you make your voice heard.

Learn to cook

Just like when you were six months old, self reliance starts with you learning to feed yourself.
Begin with something easy, like toast and eggs or a simple steak with butter and oil.
Everybody is improved as a person by learning to cook.

Chew mint before exams and while studying
It's conducive to memory and retention of information

I can't help it if your teacher doesn't allow it.
Sorry.

Never give attitude to an officer

"Thank God I was a jerk to that officer. My life is so much better now!"
\-   Nobody

**Nine out of ten celebrities are degenerate, mentally disturbed or drug addled
Don't listen to them**

That percentage is generous in my estimation.

When you get a job:
Work hard, hustle and do things right but
remember that the only place that you're
truly irreplaceable is at home

Call your mom

You'll regret it in the long run if you don't.

Write letters to people

There's something irreplaceable about a handwritten letter. People use physical objects as powerful connection points with others. It's why the Catholic church places so much reverence in holy relics and why people visit Graceland, the pyramids or the Alamo. We connect to others through the physical objects they have touched. A handwritten letter gives you the chance to both clarify your thoughts to that person and to make a real connection with that person. They live far longer in that recipient's heart than Hallmark cards, typed letters and text messages. They make you better as a person. They usually do the same to the ones you write to.

Practice meeting people

Conversation is a skill that benefits anyone and everyone around you, including yourself. Humor in particular is a strong indicator of intelligence, especially when placed in the context of good storytelling.

Making a good impression is important to a successful life so learning how to meet people and capture their attention and light up their interest is a practice worth investing time in.

The best thing about this advice is that you can do this anywhere because that's where the people are. Meet them at coffee shops, the DMV, gas stations, grocery stores, the hotel lobby, restaurants, museums and school. Pick any person out around you and strike up a conversation about anything. There's a sweet spot in between "Lovely weather" and "Did you know cows have four stomachs?" so don't be discouraged while you're struggling to get a feel for people. You'll have social anxiety, you may even be outright rejected and walked away from a time or two. But you will refine your ability to relate to people and find yourself having wonderful conversations with all kinds of new people more often. You'll make the world better; and yourself.

Read and watch the classics.

Your mind explodes when you realize that every good story has already been told a million times over. If you're going to watch a film or read a book, you might as well start with the original work that started it all. You don't have to dive right into the deep end with Shakespeare and Dante but get into the practice of cultivating a taste for the originals.

Be kind to everyone

Whether they deserve it or not.

Four primary things you need for energy: Exercise, Sunlight, Protein, Sleep

Things like coffee, energy drinks, special vitamins and medications are not necessary to an energized life. If you want natural, long term energy, use these four staples.

Pick up and take out the trash

Don't be a slob.

Tell your dad he's right

You know he is, you just don't feel ready to tell him yet.
But do it, before it's too late.

Go through your contacts once a week and give someone you haven't spoken to in a while a text or call

This is a small token of affection that can mean the world to people. You never know if your call came when a distant friend needed it the most. You never know if you're the only one to have thought of that person in months.

Stay loose
Stretch

You won't be young and limber forever. Keeping a habit of stretching will improve flexibility, blood flow, breathing, posture and countless other areas of your personal health you don't think about when you're young and invincible. I can feel my back tightening up just talking about this.

Sit down with a friend once a week and just talk
No TV, phones or other distractions
Just talk

People used to do this a lot more back in the day.
It's a lost but wonderful habit.

Don't drink until you're twenty-one

Trust me.

Don't smoke
If you do, wait 'till twenty-five

If you wait until you're twenty five, *you* decide whether or
not to make a habit out of it. If you smoke before that, the
choice is already being made *for* you. Your brain isn't fully
developed until you're twenty five. Give your brain and
your willpower a chance to fight back.
And your lungs.

Don't get a tattoo
If you do, wait 'till twenty-five

Ninety-nine times out of one hundred, that tattoo design you absolutely have to have on your bicep will seem embarrassingly stupid and poorly done ten years later. Wait until you mature before permanently marking yourself. By then you'll also be more likely to have the money and resources to do it right by a real professional; not that sketchy guy working out of a strip mall in the rough part of town.

Clean your room,
make your bed

No need to expand on Admiral McRaven or Jordan Peterson. Just do it.

Get a watch
Every adult needs a good watch

No, not that ugly smartwatch either. Get a real timepiece. It doesn't need to be expensive. It can be simple and economical. It does more for your wardrobe than you think.

Talk to yourself

No need to look like a crazy person.
But hearing our own thoughts spoken out loud can
sometimes give us a new understanding of what we're
actually feeling. What we say is just a small percentage of
what we think and feel so whatever thoughts actually
make it to spoken or written form are most likely the ones
that are dominating our mind in that moment.
Sometimes we even surprise ourselves.

Practice fasting

Catholics just read this and said, "well duh!"
Fasting does a lot on a physical, mental and spiritual level.
It helps to rid your body of toxins, burns fat, clarifies your thinking and can help in your ability to practice self discipline. It can be as frequent as an everyday intermittent fast or it can be a monthly twenty-four to seventy-two hour fast.
Either way, you'll be thankful you did. Also, that first meal to break the fast tastes a whole lot better.

When giving people bad news, be direct
Don't drag it out

Embellishing it with fluff, 'softening the blow' or 'adding context' doesn't make the news suck any less. Just tell the person what they need to hear and if they want to be reassured afterwards, do so. By dragging it out, you usually just add anxiety to the list of negative emotions they will feel. They can tell something bad is coming by you taking the long way around.

Gentlemen, get a nice suit
Ladies, get a nice dress

All you really need is one but if you can expand off that, terrific. It's irrelevant if you don't like wearing a suit or, ladies, if you can't stand wearing dresses. These are high tier pieces of clothing that are a mark and staple of the successful world. It may take some looking around to find the right one for you but having something nice in your closet will keep you from scrambling when the inevitable time you really need it happens.

Drive like everyone is an idiot who's trying to kill you

When you get out on the road, the only thing you can control is your own vehicle. It's terrifying how many people are essentially driving blind by texting, eating, playing with their dog, brushing their teeth, doing their makeup or fussing at their kids instead of driving with their full attention on the road. These are traffic fatalities waiting to happen. Don't let yourself get caught up in them.

The green light means you can **legally** go. It does **not** mean that it's **safe** to go. Look both ways even when the light is green. Double check before changing lanes and merging. Leave plenty of space between you and the car in front. Assume the cars around you are volatile with distracted drivers.

Caution is your best friend at the wheel.

Wake up early

Get up, sleepyhead.
There's only so many hours in the day.
Get to bed early so you can wake up early.

Put your phone or alarm on the other side of the room

It's easier to follow the habit from the previous page if you don't have the option of rolling over and hitting snooze. Getting up to walk and turn off the noise helps you start off moving and makes it more likely for you to stay up.

If you choose wisely, ten pieces of dress clothing can keep you looking professional all week

Black, white, gray, tan and navy provide a versatile base that go with a wide variety of other colors. Get some dark slacks, some neutral button up collared shirts and two solid pairs of dress shoes (preferably black and brown) and you can create a wide set of options to wear throughout the week.

You'll thank me later (or maybe your boss will).

Practice fixing small things in your house

Ever notice how old people tend to be much better at fixing things? There's a reason for that. They lived in an age when people had the common sense to not drop three hundred dollars every time a problem cropped up in their home. Sometimes you just have to fork over that six hundred bucks to call a plumber. But when you're bleeding money left and right on drywall, flooring, roofing, windows, painting and plumbing, your finances are going to go into the red pretty quickly. Nobody is good at patching a hole in the wall on their first try. You're going to screw up. But the more you do, the better you'll get at it until you find yourself relying on your skill rather than your wallet more often than not. And when in doubt how to fix something, ask your dad, your grandfather or good ol' Uncle YouTube to figure out how to fix that engine fan, broken fence or failed thermostat.
Everybody loves a handyman.

Learn to hunt, fish and clean an animal

Sorry vegans, this just ain't your page.
Being self reliant and able to capture, hunt and harvest
your own food does a few things for you. Firstly, it gives
you a fighting chance if things ever do go wrong with this
whole society we've built. You don't have to build a bunker
in your backyard but it never hurts to have this skill just
in case things really go south due to war, economic
collapse or logistical and infrastructure problems. If the
grocery store and restaurant are the only way you know
how to eat, you're pretty helpless to say the least.
Secondly, hunting and fishing for your meals gives you a
whole new appreciation for nature, for the wildlife we
depend on to eat and for the meals you will enjoy from
that labor. Contrary to what P.E.T.A. will tell you, hunters
typically have a much deeper appreciation for nature and
animals than your average grocery protestor.
Finally, going out to hunt and to fish gives you time away
from daily life. It distances you from some of the tedious
affairs of your world like the latest show, the most recent
news and the constant city or suburban noise that crowds
up so much of our day. Being in the woods or the shoreline
or the creek or fields lets your mind reset and fully relax.
Take advantage of that.

Talk to your grandparents and ask them as many questions as possible

They miss you.
Spend time with them while they're still around.

Set two emails
One for work and professional endeavors, the other for signups,subscriptions & accounts

It's easier to ignore that tidal wave of spam if it isn't mixed in with stuff you *have* to read.

Equip your vehicle with everything you'd need for two or three days away from home

You never know when life will call you to adventure...or when you'll forget your luggage.

Tip your servers, valets, and barbers

Anyone else is just panhandling.

Walk around barefoot often, especially on the grass

We were born barefoot for a reason.

Don't host a gathering if you're not willing to thank each person individually for coming

They drove all across town, canceled other plans, possibly got lost and probably brought gifts.
The least you can do is say 'Thanks for coming'.

Learn to shoot: gun, bow, crossbow, etc. Doesn't matter what

You can't really learn to hunt without one, can you? Also, a gun is the great equalizer when it comes to self defense, ladies. It's my firm belief that every woman should know how to shoot and own a good handgun. Learn to shoot, get your concealed handgun license and keep it in your purse out in public.
I think our society would see a **lot** less violent assaults on innocent women if they were packing heat.
Learn to shoot.

Always keep a knife or a multi tool with you

There's so many good uses for one. There will hardly come a day where you don't find some use for a blade, a pair of pliers or a file. Keep it with you and keep it clean and sharpened...just maybe not at the airport.

Keep your head up in public, especially the cities

The world is a dangerous place, but never more so than for the unobservant.

Speak with downward inflection
You're not always asking a question

You're not five years old anymore.
Your voice conveys a lot. Ending every statement on an up tone as if you're unsure just sends a message that you're clueless. Speak in a calm and matter of fact way and see how much more the world takes you seriously. When you become a parent, you'll find out quickly how much a change in tone can make a difference in how you're seen.

Learn to change a tire

It's the number one reason you'll ever be stuck on the side of the road other than maybe a dead battery or alternator (not including accidents). Don't be helpless.
Learn to change a tire. Especially you young men. If your girlfriend or wife is changing your tire, you may as well let her keep driving and leave you in the dust.

Learn to change the oil & filter on your car

Take care of your vehicle.
When you do so in a hands-on manner, it makes it much
easier.

Don't pay for landscaping service

Mow your own damn lawn.

When you're old enough, consistently invest in a slow building, stable, good dividend stock

Treat it like a plant seed. Water it weekly with manageable investment amounts that fit your budget. Watch it grow and enjoy the fruits when you're older.

Get your hair cut right

If you look like you cut your hair with a machete and styled it with a hot glue gun, you're doing something wrong. And by the way, putting strange colors in your hair doesn't substitute for a lack of personality.

Learn to read a map

Your phone has more service holes than you think. The best way to end up in the wrong place at the wrong time is to not know where the heck you're going. Between the road signs and the map, they make traveling without GPS pretty much idiot proof.

Sleep in as close to pitch blackness as you can for better sleep

I'm scared of the dark too, okay?
But you will sleep better so get over yourself.

Trouble sleeping?
Pray the Rosary

It's the Catholic in me. I can't help but suggest it. The rosary is a meditative prayer that has a powerful relaxing effect on the person reciting it, even to non-Catholics. Instructions and guides for how to pray it are abundant online and at your local Catholic parish. But if you can't bring yourself to pray the Rosary then engage in prayer and meditation on a nightly basis just as you're going to bed. There's no better way to drift off to sleep.

Make friends with the gatekeepers

Whatever you want in life is typically watched over by
someone in a position of authority over it.
A gatekeeper.
They decide who has access to it and who doesn't. The
school janitor. The assistant principal. The grocery store
manager. The front desk associate at the law firm.
Whoever it is 'guarding' the place you want to get to, it's
never a bad thing to get to know 'em. The more you follow
my earlier advice to practice talking to people, the more
success you will find when doing so with the gatekeepers.

Always keep gum or mints with you

Your breath doesn't smell too hot right now.
You need one.

Measure twice
cut once

**Listen twice
speak once**

**Always cultivate these three new habits
simultaneously:
Learn a new skill
Fast from something
Find a way to give back**

Pick one of each and work on them for sixty-seven days
and then pick a new three.

Learn to tell good stories

The best way to explain this piece of advice is by following it. Here's a little story:

When I was in college, our baseball team was sitting around in the press box during a stormy afternoon. Spring in Houston will give you plenty of opportunities to sit around inside waiting for the rain to go away. We were waiting for our coaches and those of the visiting team to decide whether our game was going to be washed out or not. To us it seemed obvious that we wouldn't play but considering that the team we were playing was from Utah, their travel expenses to Texas had to be factored in. Nonetheless, mother nature had no intention of letting us off easy. The fields were literally under water. The portable wooden mound we used for batting practice had floated from right field to center field like a raft. Trash cans floated 'downriver' across the baseball complex. We dove into water that was three feet deep and swam from the outfield fence to the press box upstairs after putting the field tarp on. I still have a few pictures on my phone as proof.

As the coaches and umpires decided amongst themselves what to do, the players waited upstairs for any updates. As we sat all around the cramped and mildewed room listening to the heavy patter of rain on the windows and aluminum bleachers outside we got restless trying to figure out how to pass the time. So one by one, we began telling stories to the group.

We told stories of ridiculous teammates we'd had, crazy people we've met, strange situations we've been in and wild accomplishments we've managed. As the evening unwound, the air began to fill with laughter as more and more players added their own insight to each story. The vibe of the room went from impatient and moody to uproarious and engaged. By the time the game was officially called off, the team had bonded through laughter and storytelling. It came at just the right time as well. After a long season, we had been just about at each other's throat by that series. Tensions were high. After that rainout, that tension had been greatly released and we played with our old team chemistry for the remainder of the season, going on to win a conference championship a few weeks later. There was a little extra magic in those last few weeks of the season and I have to believe that time in the pressbox played a significant role in that.

You have no idea how much magic you can create in people's lives when you can tell a good story and do so with intrigue, humor and wit. It may be one of our most wonderful skills in humanity and those who can express that talent are working with an incredible form of communication. Good storytellers can inspire families, communities and nations.

There's power in a good story.

On Dating

When I first wrote this book, I had all of the advice in this part ready to go and then decided not to include it.

That was a mistake.

One of the biggest problems facing our rising generations is a hesitance, hostility or misunderstanding of the dating world, what its purpose is and how to succeed in it. There's widespread confusion, reluctance, and anxiety among young people and a legion of 'experts' pumping a sewage line of bad information on them.

The results have been catastrophic.

Women follow the advice of podcasts telling them to either hate and resent all men or to give themselves away like a scrap of meat to any man who asks out of a false sense of 'empowerment'. The feminist movement embodies this 'hatred and empowerment' theme. Men are led blindly into treating women like rocks to collect and discard or are taught to resent and distrust all women as if they were ticking time bombs waiting to explode. 'Men going their own way' is a significant example of this.

In reality, men and women are made for each other. There's no great conflict or battle of the sexes. There's no need for distrust or animosity. One woman's experience doesn't dictate the life of another and one man's skill does not explain the failure of another.
Over generations there used to be some basic, common sense practices that made dating far less stressful, much more fun and wholesome for everyone involved.

These were practices passed down by grandma and grandpa and by mom and dad and supported by a culture that cherished the end result of dating: marriage.

Most of these pieces of advice are written as habits for men to practice but that does not mean that this section of the book is written for young men only. I consider the advice directed towards men to be helpful guidelines for women about what to look for in the young men they date. So ladies, pay attention too. This is a 'green flag' list to use a modern term.

For instance, if the tip tells men to "open the car door for her", then the next time a young lady who has read this passage goes on a date, she should look for a gentleman humble and respectful enough to open the door for her. The benefits of these tips are shared by men and women alike, as they have for hundreds of years. While some of the directions have been updated to match the technology of the times, the thrust of each idea is from an older and more successful time concerning the world of relationships.

Here are a handful of those long-lost practices.

Walk on the street side

Gentlemen, the purpose of a man in the relationship is to
be a provider and protector. When you walk with a lady on
a sidewalk or boardwalk you display, in a small way, that
you mean to keep her safe by walking in between her and
potential harm. In this case, walking on the street side
puts you in between her and the dangers of passing cars.
On a boardwalk, staying on the water side places you in
between her and possibly falling in the water.
It's a small gesture but it sends an important message:
I want to keep you safe.

Open every door for her

This is another token gesture that sends an important
message: I want to *serve* you.
You are telling a young lady that you are willing to clear
the path so that hers is easier to walk. You are not saying
that she is *incapable* of opening a door or that she *needs*
you to open a door.
Service is not always based on need. Neither is care.
This is affection in the form of service.

Pull out her chair for her

The same concept for the previous tip also applies to this one. *Service* and *care*. Two staples of a high value *gentleman.*

Rise from your seat when she arrives or leaves

This tip sends a message seen around the world during royal banquets, diplomatic meetings and military events: *Respect.*

It is a common custom across many cultures to rise from your seat as a sign of respect when a guest of honor rises from or arrives at theirs. What you are showing when you do this is that you have a respect to acknowledge her presence and her departure. It is insulting to remain seated while your date stands. It shows laziness, a sense of superiority and a lack of class. Be better.

Rise from your seat when she arrives or leaves.

Say her name often and with positivity

If a relationship is anything, it is certainly personal. And there are few things more personal to a person than their name. Speaking it deliberately is a sign of recognition. When you do this, and do it with positivity and energy in your voice, you send a message that she is someone worth thinking of, openly recognizing and being excited about. Christ tells us directly that He calls us each by name. This is meant to be a direct and personal call to each of us. The same goes for the relationship between a couple. Pet names like 'sweetheart' and 'honey' can show their affection sometimes but over time they can depersonalize who you're speaking to.

So say her name often and do so with positivity.

Cook for her

Earlier in this book we talked about the importance of
learning how to cook. This is another reason why.
Not every date night has to be at a five star steakhouse
that breaks your wallet in this economy.
You also don't have to be Chef Gordon Ramsay to impress
a woman with a good meal.
Find something she likes to eat and either go to grandma,
mom or good ol' Uncle YouTube to learn how to shop for
it, prepare it, cook it and serve it.
It's a lot easier than you think and it gives the evening a
much finer touch when you put your own labor and care
into a meal she enjoys.

Date for *values* first
Don't waste time

This will be longest passage of 'On Dating' and with good reason:
Dating has one end goal and one end goal only: **Marriage**

For some readers, that may make your head spin or outright explode. It's a crazy new idea that's only several thousand years old. Courtship has only ever been designed to lead to marriage.
That doesn't mean that once you begin to date someone, you're locked in for life or that you have to start picking out furniture and group insurance.
All it means is that when you are dating someone, the goal isn't to find someone to 'live with', 'spend your time with', 'be intimate with', 'rebound with' or be a 'business partner' with.
These are all things a good spouse can be but they are not end goals. Intimacy is important, gentlemen, but a woman is not a piece of meat to satisfy your hunger. Spending time with someone is important, ladies, but a man does not need to share every music, movie, show and store preference as you. (By the way, if you're consulting astrology to decide your boyfriend or girlfriend, you may need to soak your head in ice water for a few minutes and try to reboot your brain).
Each person you date (and hopefully that's not *too* many) is meant to be driven by a desire to find out if the two of you could spend the rest of your lives together on a solid foundation of faith, love and the possibility of raising a family. By the way, very few young people think they will ever want kids. That's not unusual. But before you decide to make a vow of childlessness, you may want to consider that your views on children and a family and a legacy will

change as you mature. Keep in mind, you once loved coloring books, Baby Shark and Kids Bop. Your views mature over time.

Anyway, when you are searching for a potential wife or husband, it's important to keep a few facts in mind. The first is that, more often than not, issues of trust, priorities, the *manner* of solving conflicts, substance abuse and children will be major factors in divorce. In other words, a clash of *values* is at the source. This means that sharing a faith and belief system is the single most *crucial* aspect to dating successfully.

(To date *successfully* means to make it all the way to a long lasting marriage, <u>not</u> to date a bunch of people)

Read that again!!

This is why arranged marriages, particularly in the Jewish, Muslim and Indian cultures, have such impressive numbers of successful marriages despite the fact that the courtship phase of the relationship is almost nonexistent. The couple is matched based on their faith, their family values and their culture matching up. Beyond that their interests and passions can be a world apart but they are determined to love each other and live fulfilling lives together as man and wife.

You don't need to go to football games together, listen to all the same music or run in the exact same friend circles. What you do need is to have the same beliefs in God, commitment to prayer, openness to marriage and children and the kind of community you wish to be a part of. Matching on these levels will give you statistical teflon against all other trials and mismatches life may throw at you.

Also, men, you'll display more masculine maturity and discipline when you search for the *values* in a woman rather than one misleading but alluring aspect of her.

Finally, once you *have* begun to date seriously for values, you may be lulled into a sense of complacency and desire to make absolutely sure that she is 'the one'. You've seen so much good in her and you are almost certain that she's the girl you want to spend the rest of your life with.
BUT!
She has a couple of quirks that maybe you're not a fan of.
Or maybe her family isn't quite like yours.
Or maybe you don't feel ready financially.
Or maybe the last fight y'all had gave you a suspicion that maybe she still needs to work a bit on conflict resolution.
I'll make this simple for you: Get over yourself.

Get your head out of the clouds and realize that you will *never* know one hundred percent if a girl is 'The One' before you marry her. She's not Neo, okay?
What *truly* makes a girl 'the one' is your *choice* to love her and spend the rest of your life together. I have a ratio I like to give friends; you can only be up to ninety percent certain that she's the one. What gets you the *remaining* ten percent is you *choosing* her. Making the leap closes that gap and gives you the extra determination to ensure that you live a fruitful and fulfilling life as her provider and protector.
If you spend years dating, all you are doing is wasting her time, wasting her life and showing her that you will always have doubt and distrust in her. It's a horrible and dishonoring message to give to a young lady that can shatter her perception of herself.
Date for values. Don't waste time.

Be kind and courteous
but never a pushover

There's no excuse to not be considerate but have your own
opinions. If you disagree with her about something, speak
up in a tactful and loving way. She needs to know you care
about her but she also needs to know you have a spine.
You can't be her protector if you buckle at any
disagreement.

Agreeing with everything she says won't make her like you more

This is mostly a problem with younger teens when they are first exploring ways to get a girl to like them. They see that a girl lights up about a certain topic and they get scared to put a damper on that enthusiasm by telling her they don't think the same way or enjoy that same thing. You can show her you appreciate her opinions and views without sharing them exactly.

Speak up for yourself. Be an individual.

If she wanted to date the same person, she'd go out with a mirror.

Avoid someone who doesn't respect your family

You don't have to like someone's family. But respecting the family is respecting the person by extension. Moms and Dads across history have always had a sixth sense with this. Disrespect of family is a *huge* red flag and if it is ever shown, needs to be immediately addressed and resolved before the relationship goes any further.

Don't date someone who can't dress modestly

This is another message of respect that is sent before a person even opens their mouth. Dressing modestly doesn't have to mean modern women walking around in Victorian era dresses or men in powdered wigs and knickers. But the way young people dress now just shows a lack of class. To speak more colloquially, they dress like trash.

Men who look like they just crawled out of bed ten minutes before meeting or have their shirt unbuttoned halfway down and are showing their butt crack should be turned down flat in any advance they make on a young woman.

Women who dress with more skin showing than swimsuit models leave nothing to the imagination and send a message that the only thing they have to offer is displayed out in the open for any other guy to enjoy.

Anyone who is okay with communicating to the world that they are just a piece of flesh that will go to the highest bidder is not worth your time and most likely does not share your values.

Learn to dance

You don't need to have the moves like Jagger. Just be
willing to go out on the dance floor and look a *little* bit
better than a drugged up stork having a seizure.
Have fun with it. She certainly will.

Learn to fight

There is a difference between a dangerous man and a man
who is a danger to others.
A dangerous man, one who can fight and fight well, has
the option to use violence to protect someone he cares for.
Martial arts are great at understanding this concept.
A man who is a danger to others, has no other option than
to placate a threat. The option to subdue a threat to
someone he cares for isn't even on the table.
A good man should be *capable* of violence and have the *self
discipline* to keep it tucked away until the moment leaves
no other alternative. He is more likely to be calm during
times of chaos because he always has that option of
combat training if things go from worse to worst.
Men are providers. They are also *protectors.*
Learn to fight.

Clearly communicate what you want

Be direct.
Don't expect someone to read your mind no matter how
well they know you.

If you want to date a quality woman become a quality man *first*

You can't catch a tiger with a shoelace.
If you want to be with a woman who has values, class and
virtue, you need the same values, class and virtue yourself.
You need the right tools for the right job.
Expect more of yourself before raising your expectations
of anyone, including in the dating world.

Be kind to your mother and sisters

Your girlfriend is watching how you treat the women in
your life.
Ladies, if he treats his mom poorly, there's no reason he
won't treat you just the same. Avoid men who cannot
show courtesy and care to any woman they interact with.

Acknowledge her around your friends

You may take some razzing from your friends afterwards but a lady wants to feel valued regardless of who you are with at the moment. Include her in conversations and let her be a part of what you're doing.
She doesn't need to go on your hunting trips or tag along in the locker room but she should be a real part of your life, not just an object to put on your shelf when you're not using it.

Make a good impression with her parents

Make eye contact when speaking to both mom and dad.
Speak clearly and decisively.
Shake her dad's hand like a man; firm.
Be confident and courteous.
Don't hide behind your date and actually talk to them.

Don't swear in front of her

This one is particularly hard for me. I just can't seem to
shake those four letter words.
Even if she knows you cuss, holding your tongue in front
of her shows that you have a respect for her and an ability
to be more disciplined when you're with her. You show her
that she is of a high enough value to you to behave
differently than when you are just with your friends.
Ladies, curbing your language in front of him shows that
you have class and dignity. He'll be more willing to hold
himself to a higher standard for you if you show this one
small point of restraint.

Don't tolerate crass behavior in front of her

This follows the same logic as restraining your language. No matter how funny fart jokes, cursing, or wild and raucous antics are among your friends, a little restraint goes a long way in her seeing you as a man and not a boy. You can always enjoy that stuff with your friends.

Don't 'blow it out' for holidays
Your time is more valuable to a quality woman than trinkets

Everybody speaks their own love language and to some, 'Gift Giving' may be theirs. If that is the case for your special someone, then by all means, tokens of affection like a small necklace or sweater can't hurt. But it simply isn't sustainable, practical or effective to buy the affection of someone, no matter who it is.
Remember that your time is one of the most valuable things you can give to a good woman who cares about you.

Plan dates
Don't just 'wing it'

There's nothing wrong with a little adventure from time to time. Especially while you're young and before life picks up speed on you, it can be a fun thing to grab your girlfriend and head out across the state or country to explore the world.

But having a plan will keep you from getting her into some regrettable situations. Remember part of your job is protector. You can't do that if you're such a logistical mess that even *you* don't know what the heck you're doing.

Be decisive but also open to her opinion

It's not always easy.
It helps if you just trust in God and do your best to follow
that calling.

Ask her questions about herself and try to remember the answers

I'm sure you're very interesting and all but showing interest in *her* will go a lot farther than talking about *you* all day.
Try it.

Take note when she shows an interest in something

This is another one I struggle with from time to time. Anytime a birthday, Christmas or other gift themed holiday comes around, most guys look completely lost and end up getting their girlfriend or wife a gift that says something like, 'I *really* haven't been paying attention to you all year."
Send a different message. Anytime she speaks positively about something, whether it's a movie coming out, a skirt at the mall, a tourist destination or a musician coming to town, make a note of it immediately and be ready to pounce on an opportunity for a gift or date idea.

Take her to church

You can't exactly share values if you're not willing to go
where those values begin.
Church may even be the best place to find a good young
woman to date in the first place.
It's certainly better than a club.

Learn her love language

There's a best selling book by Gary Chapman called *The Five Love Languages* published in 1992.
I'll let you read through its lessons yourself but one of the points of the book is that we all express and receive affection in a variety of ways. The general ways we do so are :
Words of Affirmation
Acts of Service
Physical Touch
Quality Time
Gift Giving
Learning which of these expressions makes your girlfriend feel the most appreciated and cared for will go a long way in your relationship. It will keep you from feeling like you do countless things to show her you care but still disappoint her. Perhaps you're just not speaking the same language.
A note of caution:
All of these languages are equally important. The key to using this information effectively is understanding the timing and frequency of each.

Be faithful
Trust is easily broken and
nearly impossible to restore

If you can't follow this one, I really can't help you.

Just listen
You don't always need an answer

There will be times when she needs your advice or input on something.
Other times, she just needs to feel heard. Having her thoughts just race around her head like a hornets nest can drive her crazy. She needs some help letting it out for a bit. Just be patient, listen and ask questions when appropriate.
Listen.

Ninety percent of communication is nonverbal

This doesn't let you off the hook to not speak clearly
about what you want as I've already explained.
But be mindful of how you express yourself in your body
language and facial expressions. Even if you are saying the
right words, rolling your eyes, sighing, crossing your arms
or pacing frantically can send a message that you are
insincere or dismissive.
She's not just listening to what you say. She's paying close
attention to how you react or respond. Be mindful of what
you are communicating without ever opening your
mouth.

Stay fit

Buying clothes for brands and logos is a lazy form of fashion. If you *really* want to look your best and not have to pay through the nose to do it, stay in good shape and buy clothes that fit.

Gentlemen...your *hair*...please

Hair is the make up for men. Take it seriously.
As I said earlier in this book, get your hair cut right.
Wash it.
Condition it.
Style it like you have some sense.

**Confidence is attractive
Arrogance is repulsive**

Raising your voice never helps

Remain calm no matter how heated a disagreement or fight may become. Always ask yourself, "Am I helping to restore peace right now or am I adding to the noise?" Keep your pride in check and your voice down.

Let her see you pray

Your faith is at the core of your character. Whatever you believe, it's the center of everything else you have an opinion or viewpoint of.
There's nothing to be self conscious of by praying in front of your date. There *is* something to be ashamed of by hiding the most important thing about you from someone you're interested in.

Godspeed

Reading a book on how to improve your life is one thing. Taking action to *make* it better is another. I've read many books in my life concerning the path to a better life mentally, spiritually and physically. But I can also be stubborn, intellectually lazy, impatient and absent minded. Much of the advice I've been given has gone in one ear and out the other.

That is to my own detriment.

Advice is only as effective as the person receiving it. My biggest prayer is that you find your way along God's path for you. If this book does anything, I hope it helps with that. None of my ideas are new. They are all borrowed from better, sharper and more established minds than mine. All I did was try to learn from them and simplify their ideas into a format that even people who hate reading are willing to sit down and digest. The useful thing about this book is that it's small and light enough that you can tuck it into your back pocket or throw it in your bag or car and take it with you whenever you need that reminder to write a letter, enjoy some quiet, be quick to show positive reactions or not to burn bridges.

We all need these little reminders in our lives. Say a little prayer for me because I need them quite often.

God bless you!

Mr. H

Acknowledgments

Among my many flaws is the inability to complete any project I start. I get outlandish ideas in my head and immediately start working on a way to make these monsters come to life. Unfortunately for me, (and fortunately for the world) most of these ideas never see daylight because I get too distracted, too busy or on rare occasions, common sense gets the better of me.
This book is one exception.

Thank you to my parents who gave me a love of reading and literature. I grew up as a fortunate kid who lived in a home covered with bookshelves. I truly believe that being surrounded by books all of my life played a huge role in my love for literature.

Thank you to my wife for hearing all of my ideas, the good, the bad and the absolutely horrendous. Most of them fall into category three. Thank you for watching the kids so many days as I was trying to bring this monster to life as kids were running around the house like wild savages.

The idea for this book first came from Glen Fucik, a fellow teacher and coach who has his students take a new composition notebook at the beginning of the year for eighth grade Health. Each class, he has them write down a useful piece of advice that they can apply to their lives as they grow up into young men. He calls it their 'Golden Nugget' book. I always loved that. I don't think this book has half as many lumps of gold in it as Glen's does by the end of each school year but I hope this book does the trick for a few kids.

Michael Berry, a radio host out of Houston, Texas, has established an informal tradition around graduation time of having his callers give pieces of advice to the younger men and women entering the real world. That always stuck with me. He also expresses the idea that 'if it is meant to be, it's up to me". I've always loved that. Thank's Michael. Love your show.

My father in law, Richard, gave me some practical advice when reviewing this manuscript and he's always been a creative force in his own right. He gets ideas in his head and then works tirelessly to make them into a reality. The difference is that he actually *finishes* his endeavors. He's inspired me to do a better job finishing my own. I'm hoping this is the first of many.

My lifelong friend and teammate Samm Wiggins Jr. played a huge role in helping me come up with some of the mental frameworks and tips in life that ended up being used in this book. Our long talks over cigars every other week have not only helped to keep my head on straight but also helped me to think critically about what I believe and what I think is actually necessary to succeed in life. He's always supported me in my pursuit of this book. I can't thank him enough for that.

Finally, I'd like to thank each of the students that I have taught these past years. This was for y'all. The letters I wrote to each of you made me realize how much I truly wanted to say. God has such incredible plans for each of you if you're only willing to walk the path He laid out. You have everything you need to do so and I hope this book provides a little food for thought on that journey. If you take nothing else from all the lessons you got from Mr. H, just remember that God is *real* and that He *loves* you.

About the Author

Mr. H. is a Catholic husband and father of four children. He's a graduate of Houston Christian University and is the best selling author of two books, both published in Mrs. Bauer's second grade English class. They sold one copy each; to mom and dad. He even made the illustrations on his own. They are works of high art and literature. That means he's a big time author **and** illustrator so you should listen to what he says. He lives in Missouri City, Texas with his family and is an Art and P.E. teacher when he's not writing.

If you ever see him in public you must approach him with the appropriate greeting which is, "You must be Mr. H, the best selling author of *Pete and the Pachycephalosaurus*! I'm so honored to meet you!" If your greeting is accepted by him, you may approach further and ask for an autograph.

If he accepts, you must provide your own pen (no ballpoint pens allowed) and paper. You must stand five feet away and be sure not to breathe on him. Your air cannot contaminate the space of a best selling author. Once you receive your autograph, you must promptly walk away. No photos are allowed to be taken. Now you can brag to your friends that you had the privilege of speaking to a second grade best selling author **and** getting his priceless autograph. You are one of the lucky few to receive this privilege.

Now go buy another copy of this book.